AN INTRODUCTION TO
MENTAL HEALTH

Sara Miller McCune founded SAGE Publishing in 1965 to support the dissemination of usable knowledge and educate a global community. SAGE publishes more than 1000 journals and over 800 new books each year, spanning a wide range of subject areas. Our growing selection of library products includes archives, data, case studies and video. SAGE remains majority owned by our founder and after her lifetime will become owned by a charitable trust that secures the company's continued independence.

Los Angeles | London | New Delhi | Singapore | Washington DC | Melbourne

JO AUGUSTUS, JUSTINE BOLD
AND BRIONY WILLIAMS

AN INTRODUCTION TO
MENTAL HEALTH

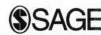

Los Angeles | London | New Delhi
Singapore | Washington DC | Melbourne

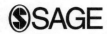

Los Angeles | London | New Delhi
Singapore | Washington DC | Melbourne

SAGE Publications Ltd
1 Oliver's Yard
55 City Road
London EC1Y 1SP

SAGE Publications Inc.
2455 Teller Road
Thousand Oaks, California 91320

SAGE Publications India Pvt Ltd
B 1/I 1 Mohan Cooperative Industrial Area
Mathura Road
New Delhi 110 044

SAGE Publications Asia-Pacific Pte Ltd
3 Church Street
#10-04 Samsung Hub
Singapore 049483

Editor: Alex Clabburn
Assistant editor: Jade Grogan
Production editor: Caroline Watson
Project manager: Swales & Willis Ltd, Exeter, Devon
Marketing manager: George Kimble
Cover design: Wendy Scott
Typeset by: C&M Digitals (P) Ltd, Chennai, India
Printed in the UK

Library of Congress Control Number: 2018947285

British Library Cataloguing in Publication data

A catalogue record for this book is available from the
British Library

ISBN 978-1-5264-2362-7
ISBN 978-1-5264-2363-4 (pbk)

At SAGE we take sustainability seriously. Most of our products are printed in the UK using FSC papers and
boards. When we print overseas we ensure sustainable papers are used as measured by the PREPS grading
system. We undertake an annual audit to monitor our sustainability.

Depression is a deafening drum, hope is in the silent echo
Jo Augustus

CONTENTS

ABOUT THE AUTHORS

Jo Augustus is a senior lecturer at the University of Worcester in the UK in the School of Allied Health and Community. She works as course leader on the Foundation Degree in Mental Health. She joined the university after 10 years working in the NHS in the UK and the independent sector, providing individual and group-based psychological interventions. She has special interests in the treatment of post-traumatic stress disorder, mood disorders, generalised anxiety disorder, low self-esteem, obsessive-compulsive disorder, binge eating disorder and bulimia. Post qualification she has completed training courses in third-wave therapies, including acceptance and commitment therapy (ACT) and mindfulness.

Justine Bold is a senior lecturer at the University of Worcester in the UK in the School of Allied Health and Community. She has worked for over 10 years on nutrition postgraduate programmes. She is researching a PhD at the University of South Wales related to the experience of illness and part of this has involved the collection of service user narratives. At Worcester, she was involved in the SHAPE project for 3 years, working with patients with severe mental health problems including psychosis, schizophrenia and bipolar disorder. She has also worked in the private sector as a nutritional therapy practitioner with clients experiencing depression and anxiety disorders.

Briony Williams is a principal lecturer at the University of Worcester in the UK and Head of the Department of Paramedic Science and Physician Associates. She qualified as an occupational therapist in 1981. Her main area of clinical experience has been in community mental health and substance misuse services throughout the UK. She has been an educator since 1999 and held a number of roles including admissions tutor for occupational therapy, programme lead for foundation degrees and lead for mental health strategy. She has a special interest in helping students to integrate theory and practice learning. Prior to working at the University of Worcester she taught on the undergraduate occupational therapy programme at Coventry University.

ACKNOWLEDGEMENTS

Jo Augustus (née Fear) – I am indebted to my wonderful husband Martin Augustus, whose love and support has carried me forward and has made all of this possible. Thank you to my amazing Mum and Dad, Tina and Nick Fear whose inspiration and wisdom inspired me to write from a young age. With thanks to my super brother Nathan Fear for being there, his wife Becky, my nephew Ieuan and niece Ffion Fear. My wonderful best friends for your love and belief in the possibilities of the unknown: Helen Piper-Windus, Marylin Winter, Beth White, Joanne Adams, Rachel Cooper, Sarah Greer, Iwona Wyprzal, Jacqui and Brian Inglis, Lizzie Harris, Barry Durkin and Shelley Limbrick. Thank you all for being there and quietly encouraging me.

Thank you also to my amazing academic colleagues, for helping me find the time and space to write, in particular to: Becka Weston for your friendship, support and laughter that has guided me through; Lisa Mauro-Bracken and Dawn Goodall for all your endless support and encouragement that has empowered me to write; Gabriela Misca for your patience and guidance; Gill Slater for your kindness and encouragement; Pete Unwin for your support and quiet humour; Helen Nicholas for your warmth and kindness; Jo Rouse for your clarity and support; Erica Pavord for your positivity and energy.

Not forgetting my co-authors Justine Bold and Briony Williams who have supported me in this venture and enabled the concept to become a reality. Thank you to my student Jan Cowin for proofreading two chapters and your helpful feedback. To all my fantastic students at the University of Worcester, too many names to write here, I have written this for you in the hope that it will inspire you in your writing. This is the end of the beginning.

Justine Bold – I would like to thank Stuart Wyley and my parents Penny and David Bold for their ongoing love and support, and also my sons Otto and Orin for bringing so much joy into my life and for giving me both motivation and strength. I would also like to thank Jo Augustus and Briony Williams for being inspiring and understanding collaborators.

Briony Williams – I would like to say thank you to my husband Richard Williams, my sons Howard, Jonathan and Patrick and my daughter-in-law Suzanne Williams for being an amazing family. Thank you to my parents Tony and Jenny Pavord for their ongoing love and support and my wonderful and inspirational siblings Ian, Andy and Erica. Finally thank you to my aunt, Anna Pavord, for inspiring me to write. Thank you to Jo Augustus for asking me to join her to write this book. Thank you Jo and Justine for all our discussions, your patience and support with proofreading.

PUBLISHER'S ACKNOWLEDGEMENTS

The authors and publisher are grateful to the following people for their invaluable feedback on the initial proposal and draft material for the book. The book is richer for having had your input.

Jeremy Dixon, University of Bath

Judith Skargon, University of Essex

Thomas Beary, University of Hertfordshire

Sue Barker, Cardiff University

Andy Mantell, London South Bank University

We would also like to thank the people who provided their (anonymous) voices for case studies; your experiences have helped to shape the rich examples of mental health care and practice considered throughout the book.

THIRD-PARTY MATERIAL

We are also grateful to the following third parties for their permission to reproduce the following material:

Table 4.1 Stepped-care model. Reproduced with permission under the terms of the NICE UK Open Content Licence.

Figure 5.1 Bio-psycho-social model in the context of chronic pain (Gatchel et al. 2007). Reproduced with permission of the American Psychological Association.

INTRODUCTION

JUSTINE BOLD, JO AUGUSTUS AND BRIONY WILLIAMS

It is hoped that this book will inform the professional training of the many health professionals and **practitioners** working with patients with **mental health** difficulties including social workers, mental health professionals, doctors, nurses, **occupational therapists**, **counsellors**, nutrition and CAM (complementary and alternative medicine) practitioners so helping to optimise available treatment options and improve chances of **recovery** for people affected by mental health problems.

The chapters that follow consider the factors underlying the development of mental health issues as well as providing guidance on how patients can best be diagnosed and be supported by evidence-based treatment. This book has an inter-professional focus as the three authors come from different backgrounds and disciplines; it aims to review the evidence and raise the awareness of the benefits of person-centred and integrated approaches to patient treatment and care as patient-centred care is associated with individual patient well-being (Gameiro et al. 2013). Narrative accounts from service users experiencing mental health problems have been included to provide additional insights. The authors believe that understanding the lived experience of mental health problems and key issues faced by people diagnosed with mental health problems is key for the health professionals of the future. It is hoped that greater understanding of the experience of mental health problems and treatment might help foster a more supportive environment for patients/clients that promotes recovery from **mental illness**.

Key issues around policy and ethics are also included and there are chapters on the history of mental health treatment as well as a brief guide to different approaches to diagnosis and treatment and supportive therapies. Some of these chapters have been structured using Engel's (1977) bio-psycho-social model of health, which is widely recognised as being a foundation for much of modern-day mental health clinical practice as it considers social and psychological factors not explored in traditional biomedicine. An example of how this has been used is in Chapter 1, on the history of mental health. This is considered from a biological point of view, then psychological and then a social perspective as the authors thought this a useful way to shape historical presentation, understanding, progression and links between the key areas. **Psychological well-being** is a central theme of this book in the context of promoting a recovery journey that is unique to every individual. Ryff and Singer (2006) refer to factors that constitute an individual's psychological well-being: positive relationships with others, personal mastery, autonomy, a feeling of purpose and meaning in life, personal growth and development. Thus, psychological well-being is arguably achieved by maintaining a balance between events that present both challenge and reward (Ryff and Singer 2006; Winefield et al. 2012). Diner, Oishi and Lucac (2003) develop the concept of psychological well-being to include the awareness that the individual has of their own integrity, in all aspects of their being. Thus, well-being also includes an awareness of the individual's sense of well-being.

International mental health is also explored in this book, both as a chapter and also as a theme. Through the recognition that globalisation is of great importance, the authors have drawn on a variety of international research in the hope of inspiring the reader to appreciate the possibilities of learning from international perspectives and in doing so, further developing the concept of global mental health learning communities. Finally, we very much hope this book is forward thinking in terms of its interdisciplinary focus, as it includes material on third-wave therapies and we explore the links between physical and mental health and other lifestyle and nutritional factors including coeliac disease, which can all impact upon mental health.

REFERENCES

Diner, E., Oishi, S. and Lucac, R. E. (2003) Personality, culture, and subjective well-being: emotional and cognitive evaluations of life. *Annual Review of Psychology* 54: 403–425.

Engel, G. (1977) The need for a new medical model: a challenge for biomedicine. *Science* 196: 129–136.

Gameiro, S., Verhaak, C. M., Kremer, J. A. M. and Boivin, J. (2013) Why we should talk about compliance with assisted reproductive technologies (ART): a systematic review and meta-analysis of ART compliance rates. *Human Reproduction Update* 19(2): 124–135.

Ryff, C. D. and Singer, B. (2006) Psychological well-being meaning measurement, and implications for psychotherapy research. *Psychotherapy and Psychosomatics* 65: 14–23.

Winefield, R. H., Gill, K. T., Taylor, W. A. and Pilkington, M. A. (2012) Psychological well-being and psychological distress: is it necessary to measure both? Psychology of well-being: theory. *Research and Practice* 2(3): 1–14.

1 A HISTORY OF MENTAL HEALTH

BRIONY WILLIAMS AND JUSTINE BOLD

———————————— LEARNING OBJECTIVES ————————————

After studying this chapter you will be able to:

• understand the history of **mental health** from a bio-psycho-social perspective;
• understand specific interventions that were used in the treatment of mental health conditions;
• consider how history has helped shape and develop current mental health practices.

INTRODUCTION

In the past there have been many explanations for understanding **mental illness** including possession by the devil and punishment by a god, curses of witches or wizards and also physical causes such as bad humors and an imbalance of chemicals. The ancient Greek writer Homer interpreted the 'irrational' elements in human nature as an interference by the gods. In some cultures today these explanations still exist. Psychological explanations did not emerge until fairly recently. These biological, social and psychological theories about the origins of mental illness influenced and directed the treatments and services. New treatments were generally developed because of expanding knowledge and changing societal views. However, where people were cared for (i.e. at home, in the community, hospital or in an asylum) was influenced by societal views of mental illness. Biological, psychological and social explanations gained power at different times in history and at some points in history competed for supremacy. There are still biological, psychological and social theories of the origins of mental health problems, which make the causes of mental illness difficult to understand. Modern-day psychiatry is criticised for having a primarily biological understanding of mental illness (Scull 2014). The rise in biological psychiatry is viewed by Bentall (2004) as 'owing more to politics and financial interests of drug companies than to science and evidence' (p. 173). After the Second World War there was a move by psychiatrists in America to put forward psychological explanations of mental health problems, and cures involved talking therapy

(Scull 2011). The social model that emerged from the disability movement in the late twentieth century meant that service users started to be more willing to question the opinion of professionals and be less willing to accept what they are told by **consultants**. This chapter will now explore the history of mental illness and treatment in terms of biological, social and psychological contexts.

BIOLOGICAL EXPLANATIONS

Biological theories of the origin and treatment of mental health problems are put forward by those interested in the physical workings and structures of the body. Known as the medical or biological model, it is concerned with classifying and understanding mental health problems through science, using terms such as diagnosis, prognosis and treatment. Proponents of biological theories look to understand the causes by using X-rays, brain scans and blood tests to measure chemicals in order to classify the illness (make a diagnosis). The diagnosis and the prognosis (the likely outcome) inform the treatment plan. Treatments involve medication to change body chemistry and physical interventions such as surgery and **electroconvulsive therapy (ECT)**. Some of these medical treatments have been invasive and involve unpleasant side effects. Some treatments such as ECT and prefrontal lobotomy were barbaric in their conception and delivery – done by those in power to those in distress. However some medical treatments and research have led to a much better quality of life for people living with serious mental health problems.

EARLY PHYSICAL EXPLANATIONS

Physical explanations involved humoral medicine, which started with the classical Greek physician Hippocrates (460–377 BC) and was disseminated more widely by the Roman Galen (129–216 AD). The basic idea behind humoralism was balancing fluids found in the human body; these were named the four humors and were black bile, yellow bile, blood and phlegm and they represented different qualities. The humors could be matched to different parts of the body, the four seasons and different emotional characteristics (see Table 1.1).

Table 1.1 Humors

Humor	Season	Element	Characteristics	Description
Black bile	Autumn cold and dry	Earth	Melancholic	Despondent and gloomy
Yellow bile	Summer hot and dry	Fire	Choleric	Bad tempered
Blood	Spring hot and wet	Air	Sanguine	Courageous, hopeful and amorous
Phlegm	Winter cold and wet	Water	Phlegmatic	Calm, cool and unemotional

Classical medicine in the medieval period was all about balancing these humors, by changing diet, lifestyle, occupation and climate or by administering medicine. In order to bring the body back into equilibrium, patients were given purgatives with emetics to induce vomiting, laxatives and people were bled using leeches or cupping (Macdonald 1981). This was as true for mental illness as it was for somatic diseases. So, if someone was melancholic, they suffered from an excess of black bile; if they were manic, it was either too much blood or yellow bile that was the problem. Balancing one's lifestyle, therefore, was central to one's emotional well-being (Smith 2016). The Chinese at this time had similar thoughts, believing madness was an imbalance of the primal forces of yin and yang.

BLOODLETTING

One form of treatment involved in balancing humors was bloodletting. Galen (129–200 AD) declared blood as the most dominant humor so the practice of venesection gained even greater importance (Magner 1992). There was more than one method of bloodletting, including removing blood from a blood vessel by cutting or localised methods including scarification with cupping and using leeches. Benjamin Rush, founder of the American temperance movement (Shryock 2006), also often referred to as the father of American psychiatry, was well known as an advocate of vigorous bloodletting (Garrick 2010), while Earle Pliny questioned the appropriateness of bloodletting as a treatment for mental health problems in 1854. Pliny's overall conclusion supported a trend towards a correlation between better **recovery** and less use of bloodletting procedures. Rush had a long-running feud with his college of physicians regarding his use of bloodletting, which forced him to resign (Greenstone 2010).

LOBOTOMY

Prefrontal lobotomy is intentional damage to the prefrontal lobe of the brain, which claimed to be a cure for **schizophrenia**. A lobotomy is surgery that could be seen as a combination of neurosurgery and psychiatry called psychosurgery. The origins of psychosurgery can be traced back to antiquity, with evidence of Stone Age craniotomies dating as far back as 5100 BCE (Smith 2016). Carpenter and Davies (2012) note that in searching for treatments for schizophrenia, 'prefrontal lobotomy had the broadest application and achieved a desired calming effect but at the expense of vital emotional processing and motivational qualities' (p. 1168).

ELECTROCONVULSIVE THERAPY (ECT)

ECT is a treatment that involves sending an electric current through the brain to trigger an epileptic seizure. It was first used in 1939 and is still used to relieve the symptoms of some mental health problems such as severe depression, post-natal depression, schizophrenia and sometimes **bipolar disorder**. The treatment involves applying brief but powerful shocks via two electrodes called paddles placed on the patient's forehead. Using ECT as a treatment may have been based on the knowledge that head trauma and convulsions were observed to improve mental disturbances. Hippocrates noted that malaria-induced convulsions cured some insane patients (Sabbatini 1998). In the Middle Ages some physicians observed that after a bout of fever such as the cholera epidemic in insane asylums people's mental health symptoms improved. Between 1917 and 1935 four methods for producing physiological shock were discovered and tested including malaria-induced fever, insulin-induced coma and convulsions and ECT (Pridmore 2009). ECT was considered less dangerous than the drug-induced convulsions or comas. The technique became widespread in hospitals across Europe and North America. ECT was widely used in the 1950s and 1970s and sometimes without anaesthetic and often without **consent**. Some people may experience the procedure as a punishment rather than a treatment and the main side effects are usually short term, but many people experience memory loss. Although the success of ECT in treatment of **depression** is established, people still have no understanding of the evidence of how it works (The Royal College of Psychiatrists 2013). Possibly due to the fact that it is not understood, it has received much criticism. Misgivings about ECT were highlighted in films, the most famous of which was *One Flew Over the Cuckoo's Nest* in 1975 (McDonald and Walter 2001) and near this time ECT became a target of the anti-psychiatry movement. ECT was used as a treatment for homosexuality in the 1960s, as it was considered by psychiatrists at the time to be a mental illness. However, advocates of anti-psychiatry, supportive of talking therapy, were very much against using ECT. The treatment declined in use in the 1960s and 1970s, however revived in the 1980s. In more recent times the use of a professional anaesthetist is mandatory as well as the use of muscle relaxant to make sure that the patient experiences no skeletal fractures. The Royal College of Psychiatrists (2013) reported on a survey of 7,880 clinics in England and Wales assessing outcomes for people who received ECT in 2012 and 2013. The findings were that 1,712 people changed either minimally, much or very much, there was no change in 113 people and 28 people got worse.

MEDICATION

By the late 1950s and early 1960s, new medications began to change psychiatry, starting with the discovery of the first antihistamines (effective in dealing with hay fever) in the 1940s and 1950s. These drugs provided a chemical basis from which a wide range of drugs used in psychiatry were developed. These early antihistamines often induced sleepiness and sedation. Pharmacologists and psychiatrists wondered if this sedative effect could be used to 'calm' the positive symptoms in schizophrenia (Marston 2013).

A new class of antidepressants called SSRIs (selective serotonin reuptake inhibitors) were better tolerated and medically safer than prior antidepressants. The first of these, Prozac, was released in 1987. Following this introduction new anti-psychotics were released: 'atypical neuroleptics' such as Risperdal and Zyprexa. These drugs were heavily promoted as they had apparent advantages over earlier drugs, and were widely prescribed by psychiatrists. At this time public research money strongly shifted towards neuroscience and pharmaceutical research (Klein and Glick 2014).

The National Institute of Mental Health (NIMH) invested to enhance public aware-ness of the benefits to be derived from brain research (Marston 2013). By the 1990s biological psychiatry appeared to have become the main theory and therefore treat-ment. However, public and private investment and pharmaceutical innovation decreased in the 2000s (Klein and Glick 2014). No new classes of medication psychi-atric drugs were discovered despite funding and research. The media highlighted previously unrecognised side effects of widely used medications. SSRIs were impli-cated in increased suicidal behaviour, and some patients reported severe 'discontinuation syndromes' when stopping treatment. Atypical neuroleptics were associated with a 'metabolic syndrome', which includes significant weight gain, increased diabetes risk, and other medical complications (Marston 2013). However the money spent on basic brain research led to no advancement in understanding of psychiatric aetiology, nor to new biological treatments. Pharmaceutical companies were fined repeatedly and for huge sums for promoting powerful, expensive psychi-atric medications for unapproved uses (Marston 2013).

SOCIAL THEORIES

The ancient Greek writer Homer, thought to have lived between the twelfth and eighth centuries BC, suggested that human action is caused by bodily organs, notably the brain. Plato, the Roman philosopher writing later, thought that the essence of the human body is the psyche, rendered in English as 'soul' or 'mind' (Spillane 2006). This focus on the soul continued up to and through the fifteenth century, as before this people were viewed as having souls, rather than minds. Descartes (1596–1650), writing in the seventeenth century, described the concept of mind–body dualism for the first time. He proposed that the body is a machine and that its physiology can be explained according to the principles of physics. The soul differs, having one entity and being free. Descartes (1968) concludes that he is a soul and he has a body con-tingently attached to the soul (Spillane 2010). This dualism has created boundaries between mind and body, the effects of which have lasted up to the present day. In terms of gender, women were portrayed as more closely linked to nature and less completely integrated into civilisation and the cultural order than men. This connec-tion between women and nature and natural cycles dates back to Greek mythology, with goddesses such as Persephone and Demeter being connected to the earth. The mind was generally related to men and civilisation and the body to nature and women; consequently loss of the mind was viewed as also a loss of civilisation and required the person to be controlled and protected (Lloyd 2002). It must be remem-bered that women at this time did not generally have independence, society was patriarchal and women were subject to family control as men were viewed as the rational agents and makers of order and measure.

Social models regard the wider influence of social forces as more important than other influences as causes of mental illness (Tyrer and Steinberg 2013, p. 104), seeing the person with mental health problems as a player on a big stage. There is currently a growing interest in 'recovery' in mental health policy and practice, although research has shown that many mental health service users consider that the medical model still dominates, which they see as damaging and unhelpful. The social model looks at how mental health issues are understood in society, people's personal under-standings of mental health issues, the social model of disability in relation to mental health and a possible social model of madness and distress. Some of the features of the social model are:

- being rights based and anti-discriminatory, rather than focusing narrowly on the individual;
- valuing self-management and self-support;
- a commitment to anti-oppressive practice;
- supporting race equality and cultural diversity;
- prioritising advocacy and self-advocacy;
- minimising compulsion in the psychiatric services by prioritising prevention, rapid and appropriate support and advanced directives;
- breaking the bad/mad link that continues to be a driver in mental health policy and provision;
- prioritising participation in the development, management and running of policy and services;
- equalising power relations between **service providers** and service users in services and support (Beresford 2005, p. 115).

The social model sees the labelling and **stigma** following from a medical model of mental illness as a major barrier for mental health service users (Rowntree Foundation 2018). It argues that the medicalisation of experience and social prob-lems has dominated the conceptualisation of madness and distress. The influence of psychiatry and psychiatric thinking has also had the effect of medicalising a wide range of social concerns, reframing them in diagnostic categories for 'treatment' (Newnes 2015). These range from the human effects of war, 'post-traumatic stress disorder' (PTSD) to the non-conformist and non-cooperative behaviour of children and young people, 'attention deficit hyperactivity disorder' (ADHD) (Newnes 2015). Psychiatry also encompasses violent, criminal and dangerous behaviour by the use of an increasing range of labels like 'dangerous personality disorder' and 'narcissistic personality disorder'. Case Study 1.1 explores the treatment of women diagnosed with 'menopausal mania'.

CASE STUDY 1.1: THE TREATMENT OF MENOPAUSAL MANIA, GRACE'S STORY

My third experience was in a semi-narcosis unit. That means the people were sedated to overcome their mental health problems. The women with 'menopausal mania' needed a lot of personal care as they were basically asleep all the time. The worst bit about it was that we were persuaded that this was the treatment that worked. Having since been through the menopause and not enjoyed it one bit, I cannot see how medicating all those women could have helped overcome their symptoms. Except they were asleep for a long time and by the time they were woken up properly, all their symptoms had resolved naturally.

RELIGIOUS EXPLANATIONS

Historically religion and the church were very important in people's lives and influential in the way people understood mental illness. Mental illness was for many centuries seen as possession by the devil and treatment for mental illness focused on demonology and exorcism was performed on the person who was suffering. Direct linkage between spirit-possession and madness can be found in both Jewish and Christian scripture (Islam and Campbell 2014). The origin of attributing mental illness to supernatural causes predates Islam and is found to have existed in pagan Arabia and in Ancient Greece. The causes of insanity were unknown, so supernatural phenomena were employed to explain its existence (Islam and Campbell 2014). The New Testament contains writings about people who were possessed and were given treatment by Jesus or one of the apostles using exorcism.

> When evening came, they brought to Him many who were demon-possessed; and He cast out the spirits with a word, and healed all who were ill. (Matthew 8:16)

> So his fame spread throughout all Syria, and they brought him all the sick, those afflicted with various diseases and pains, those oppressed by demons, epileptics, and paralytics, and he healed them. (Matthew 4:24)

The ability to exorcise devils was seen as a mark of divine favour or saintliness in Christian religion. There are references to exorcism in the lives of the saints and the search for examples of exorcism to support a case for canonisation (Kemp and Williams 1987). Rather than being rooted in formalistic religion, belief in the supernatural origin of mental illness may be rooted in a broader cultural context, reflecting long-held superstitions and mystical beliefs (Kapferer 2003). Evil spirits were exorcised through incantation, prayer, cajoling, threatening and even included physical torture, scourging and squeezing the evil spirits out.

TREPANNING

This is the process of making a burr hole in the skull, essentially believed to be a primitive form of craniotomy. This was carried out to release 'evil spirits' believed to be inside people suffering from mental health disorders. Thousands of trepanned skulls from the Neolithic period (c.9000–3000 BC, depending on the region) have been found from many civilisations across the world including those in Europe, South America, China and Africa (Hobert and Binello 2017), demonstrating how widespread the process was. There is evidence of new bone formation around the holes on a number of skulls indicating that some of the victims of these primitive rituals survived the procedure (Hobert and Binello 2017).

WITCHCRAFT

People died in witch-hunts across Europe in the sixteenth and seventeenth centuries. Witchcraft trials in Salem commenced with a small group of girls who saw strange things and behaved in bizarre ways and were investigated by village elders. Cotton

Mather, a church minister, investigated the behaviour of the children. Mather concluded that witchcraft, specifically that practised by an Irish washerwoman who had yelled at the children, was responsible for the children's problems. The girls accused several local women of practising witchcraft and placing curses on them. At its worst in the year 1691 about 250 people were arrested and tried for witchcraft, of these 19 were executed, 2 died in prison and 1 died of torture (Deutsch 2013). Talismans and amulets are worn as protective devices against witchcraft.

THE INCREASE IN ASYLUM PROVISION

Prior to and during the Middle Ages, people with mental health problems were taken care of at home or by their immediate community. There was no formal provision of services; people with mental health problems were a domestic responsibility dealt with by friends and family. Due to the shame and stigma attached to mental illness, many hid their mentally ill family members in cellars, caged them in pigpens, or put them under the control of servants (Porter 2002). People with mental health problems were widely abused and restrained, particularly in Christian Europe. Others were abandoned by their families and left to a life of begging and vagrancy (Porter 2002). By the end of the medieval period there was a decline in the belief of charity as a duty. The Industrial Revolution that started in the UK in 1760 was relevant in changing the way people with mental health problems were viewed. Scull (2011) suggested that the intensification of labour created by the Industrial Revolution pushed families to admit their lunatic relatives to the asylum because they were an increasing burden in an era of extreme poverty (Melling 1999).

The first mental institution in the UK was called Bedlam, in London, which was founded in 1247 for those suffering from a mental disorder. It was taken over by the Crown in 1377. It is also likely that separation from society and the segregation of people with mostly severe mental illness became more necessary as work with machines was common. The number of asylums increased after 1780 (Rogers and Pilgrim 2001). Treatments generally used in asylums included cold baths, hot candles 'cupped' to chest and back, leeching, and electrostatic shocking to jolt patients to reality. Solitary confinement (a Quaker philosophy) was considered calming and an opportunity for reflection that might lead to rational behaviour (Norris 2017). An 1808 Act authorised magistrates to build publicly funded asylums in each county and the first Lunacy Act issued in 1845 made this compulsory. Physical control of inmates appeared to be the primary concern when asylums were planned and built, with manacles in each cell attached to the walls with chains and windows recessed and barred (Norris 2017).

It is important to be aware that some people were locked away due to being inconvenient to family or through social embarrassment (for example women who got pregnant out of wedlock or were deemed to be 'inconvenient' wives). These people may not have initially been mentally ill, but may have developed mental health problems as a result of their institutionalisation. Moreover, financial hardship was commonplace and some who were admitted to the asylum may have been poor rather than mentally ill. The local poor law receiving officer was the first port of call for those in need. One of three solutions would be considered, 'outdoor relief', usually a small amount of money, transfer to the workhouse, or transfer to the county asylum. The first option was very rarely offered and the majority of the time the poor would be sent to the workhouse (Bartlett 1998, p. 422), but some may have been transferred to the asylum. Described as a 'sham lunatic', an individual faked insanity in order to be kept in the safety of a lunatic asylum or the workhouse in the absence of a stable residence of their own.

Law and mental health policy focused on the living conditions in the asylums and the 1828 Madhouse Act introduced a system of licensing and visits to check conditions.

There were other reasons for being admitted, these included alcoholism, financial issues and shock. A handbook published in the Eugenics Review in 1912 (Lidbetter 1912, p. 26), states 'one out of every five inmates of lunatic asylums have "lost their reason" through drink ... altering the brain substance, and producing insanity', and that 'the dreadful disease known as epilepsy, often comes to the children of drinkers'. Dr Campbell working at the Garlands Hospital identified that the most 'likely cause of insanity was mental shock or worry from money losses'. By the end of the nineteenth century, the county asylum was seen by people as the place for the insane to be. By the time the 1845 County Asylums Act was passed, less than 5,000 patients were housed in asylums (Cherry 2003, p. 10) but by 1900 this number had increased to around 100,000 (Bynum, Porter and Shepherd 1988, p. 2). In the 1960s mental health provision changed, institutions were closed and care moved again into the community.

Interestingly, as Peter describes in Case Study 1.2, it was social history that influenced his decision to train as a social worker.

CASE STUDY 1.2: SOCIAL HISTORY AS AN INFLUENTIAL FACTOR IN CAREER CHOICE, PETER'S STORY

As an undergraduate, I became interested in theories of institutionalisation, particularly Goffman's work on asylums in the United States and Townsend's work on old people's homes in the UK. These works haunted me as I began a career as a social worker and became 'part of the system' that continued to place individuals in large-scale institutions, without any thought for personalisation.

The works of Laing and Szasz also stayed with me and I still lean towards a definition of most mental ill health as being on a normative spectrum – 'problems in living' – rather than states of mind that require some form of intervention by professionals. The all-pervasiveness of media imagery and social media models of personal and familial 'norms' are very damaging these days to individuals who struggle to find fulfilment in life. I wish there were a significant 'counter movement' that provided all ages with realistic aspirations regarding personal growth, relationships, family and career.

I have always been associated with the voice of service users and carers and welcome the radical, 'madness' views that some of these groups promote. My biggest regret is that I did not become more active politically in my early career, and I would urge all mental health professionals to become political and unionised. When we have decent levels of health and social care services, then we will all enjoy better mental health – service users, carers and professionals alike.

PSYCHOLOGICAL EXPLANATIONS

Sigmund Freud questioned the relationship between organic sources of madness and the psychological causes of mental illness. Freud and his followers played an important role in listening and trying to understand the complexity of the history of people with mental health problems. Breuer (1842–1925) was an Austrian physician and Janet (1859–1947) was a French neurologist, psychologist and philosopher. Works by these pioneers represented a departure from the traditional view that mental illness and unexplained medical disease were the result of divine retribution or demonic possession. Freud began the psychoanalysis movement, which accounted for the widest range of mental states as potentially leading to psychic pain without direct organic cause. He observed patients of the French neurologist, Charcot, and formulated that some of their behaviour had its roots in trauma rather than a physical biological disease. Breuer developed the cathartic method in the 1880s and he and Freud wrote together in 1895 about the treatment of hysteria. Janet published several texts on the importance of the unconscious from 1889 onwards, however Freud expanded this theory publishing theories on the unconscious roots of mental disorders that could not be explained medically, which he termed psycho-neuroses. Freud developed psychoanalysis to treat these 'neurotic' patients. It could be said that these men developed the principles of what later became talking therapies and established the significance of early adverse childhood experiences and trauma.

The First World War and the impact of shell shock, now called post-traumatic stress disorder, on servicemen blurred the distinction between neurosis and insanity. Many shell-shocked ex-servicemen were transferred to asylums. For the first time neurosis as well as psychosis became a focus of interest to psychiatrists.

THE PSYCHOANALYTICAL INFLUENCES

Psychoanalysis is mostly concerned with our inner world, suggesting it has a powerful influence on how we feel and think so therefore how we behave. Our inner world is partly conscious and mostly unconscious. It is made up of memories, feelings, beliefs and fantasies (Howard 2011). Freud suggested that there are three causes for mental distress:

- The *real world*: which includes traumatic events like crime, accidents and disasters.
- The *id*: the instinctual feelings that demand fulfilment.
- The *super ego*: when we are fearful of being punished for a moral transgression.

In Freud's view the amount of psychic energy is limited and must be shared between all three parts of the personality: the id, ego and superego; this explains why in mental distress too much energy is being used up with the ego trying to deal with unresolved conflicts. A healthy individual is able to resolve conflicts as they arise and therefore keep psychic energy for the ego to be able to develop and interact with the environment. Freud also proposed that children go through a series of psychosexual stages focused on different parts of the body. He suggested if a child does not work through a stage they become stuck at this stage of development and their personality becomes dominated by it, and the following stage cannot commence until the previous one has been negotiated. This theory may support the development of personality disorders, which are understood to develop when trauma interferes with the development of a child's personality.

TREATMENT THROUGH LSD

Freudian psychoanalysts viewed LSD as the ideal tool to reach the 'realms of the human unconscious'. Psychologists employed LSD as a tool in therapy, hoping to delve into suppressed memories and elicit revelatory experiences that could alter behaviour and cure pathology (Jacobs 2008). Psychedelics have been used by shamans and medicine men since ancient times, as a way to gain access to the spirit world. Psychedelics grow naturally in seeds, mushrooms, cacti, bark and roots of various plants. Concerns about the long-term effects of LSD led to laws restricting its use.

SHELLSHOCK TO POST-TRAUMATIC STRESS DISORDER (PTSD)

The Great Wars of the twentieth century and the lasting effects servicemen experienced led to the emergence of military psychiatry as a discipline and have over the years contributed to a greater understanding of trauma. PTSD was defined in the 1980s (McKenzie 2012); prior to this trauma associated with war and fighting had different names. In the First World War (1914–1918) it was referred to as shellshock or neurasthenia, in the Second World War (1939–1945) it was known as combat fatigue (McKenzie 2012).

In the First World War, initial treatments included ether and chloroform anaesthetics or electrical treatments (McKenzie 2012) and there was an emphasis on getting soldiers back to active duty as quickly as possible. In 1915 'forward psychiatry' was developed by the French and by 1918 the British also had forward psychiatry units. The acronym 'PIE' is used in forward psychiatry; it stands for proximity to battle, immediacy, and expectation of recovery (Jones and Wessely 2003). In the First World War, camps were set up near the front line and aggressive treatments such as electrotherapy were sometimes used to get soldiers back to the war (Tatu and Bogousslavsky 2014). While the majority of service personnel returned to the fighting, it is documented that some soldiers who refused to go back to fight were accused of malingering and tried by court martial and sentenced to death (Tatu and Bogousslavsky 2014). Around 1918, psychodynamic methods inspired by Freud started to be used in favour of the more aggressive treatments (McKenzie 2012). Even so, it has been questioned whether these early approaches serviced the needs of the military more than the needs of traumatised service personnel. By the Second World War in the 1940s treatments included barbiturates (McKenzie 2012) but seem to have remained largely similar to those used in the First World War. Hence academics have questioned whether lessons learnt from the First World War were actually applied at all in the Second World War (Rae 2007). It is fair to say that both treatments and understanding have progressed considerably since then, and current UK clinical guidance (NICE 2005) recommends both **cognitive behavioural therapy** and antidepressants for PTSD associated with combat.

BEHAVIOURAL INFLUENCES

The behavioural model put forward in the 1920s suggests that behaviour, autonomic responses, thoughts and feelings are linked and are all important mental processes and that thoughts and feelings are altered by changes in behaviour. The emphasis in this model is on behaviour because it is easily observed, measured and modified. Behaviour is learned when it is reinforced, therefore it is proposed we can also learn maladaptive behaviours. Classical conditioning was researched by Pavlov in 1897, who presented food to dogs at the same time as a sound, so the dogs gradually associated the sound with food and eventually salivated when they heard the sound. This model shows how everyday sounds and smells can be turned into traumatic stimuli because they are associated with a traumatic event (Gibson 2006). Skinner working in 1936 proposed that reward and punishment were important in strengthening and weakening behaviour. If we are rewarded when performing a behaviour we are likely to repeat that behaviour, if we are punished we will avoid the behaviour. If punishment is stopped when we perform a behaviour we are more likely to reproduce the behaviour. The behavioural model is criticised as focusing on symptoms and ignoring the cause.

COGNITIVE BEHAVIOURAL MODEL

The cognitive behavioural model was developed in the 1970s. At the time there was increasing dissatisfaction with **behavioural therapy**, which was seen as reductionist. Cognitive behavioural therapy was influenced by two clinicians, Albert Ellis and Aaron Beck. Beck developed the cognitive model, which suggests people have a schemata, which could be seen as a framework holding rigid long-lasting views about themselves, the world and other people. Due to their schemata people create rules about how to behave. Some of these rules are maladaptive and although understandable at the time of creation can cause problems later in life during adulthood. A critical incident or stressful life event can fire up the maladaptive rules and increase negative automatic thoughts and symptoms of **anxiety** and depression (Beck 1976).

COMMUNITY CARE

Services started shifting away from the asylum after the First World War and outpatients and services in the community were set up. Deinstitutionalisation involved moving care and treatment of people with mental health problems from the asylum into community-based settings. The policy of closing the asylums began the challenges made to the power of psychiatry and psychiatric institutions that were a feature of the 1960s (Cummings 2012). Other reasons may include the development and increased use of major tranquilisers. However, Scull (1977) believes it was only due to the cost of running large institutions and keeping people in hospital. At the start of the process of moving to community care, in the 1950s asylums housed approximately 154,000 people, in the 1970s the number was 100,000 and by the end of the process the asylums had all closed (Gilbert et al. 2014). Under the 1962 Hospital Plan, acute psychiatric inpatient services were developed on district general hospital sites, local authorities were developing **community mental health teams** and there was an increased outpatient role. However, as the author (BW) recollects, working in a district hospital in the early 1980s the number of acute psychiatric inpatient beds in the district hospitals was significantly higher than the number today.

The 1980s brought changes to the management structure and systems in the National Health Service (NHS). Roy Griffiths believed 'that a small, strong general management body is necessary at the centre of the NHS' (Taylor 1984). Following this a proposal was put forward for a fundamental restructuring of the NHS structure and a reorganising of duties and responsibilities, accountability and control. Griffiths' ideas involved a new NHS management board, at arm's length from the secretary of state and civil servants, and identifying general managers with overall responsibility for performance and budgets at district health authorities and hospital units. For the first time in its existence the NHS had managers leading their hospitals. In 1997 Labour issued the 'new NHS – modern, dependable,' which built on current trends with better communication within the service, GP out-of-hours services increasingly using nurses to assess emergency calls, NHS Direct (the new nurse-led helpline) and a focus on quality with new national supervisory bodies. Labour established a National Institute for Clinical Excellence to investigate and approve cost-effective pharmaceuticals and interventions for use in the NHS and a Commission for Health Improvement (later the Healthcare Commission) to check what was happening. As part of the programme to modernise and reform the NHS, the Labour Government set up National Service Frameworks (NSFs) in order to improve patient care and reduce inequalities in a series of identified priority areas (Gilbert et al. 2014). The National Service Framework for Mental Health emerged because of pressure to reform community mental health care. Media coverage of a series of high-profile adverse events involving people with mental illness contributed to a public perception that community care had failed (Kings Fund 2014). The incorporation of the European Convention on Human Rights into UK law was a further reason to reform mental health legislation. Over several decades large mental health hospitals were closing and being replaced by community psychiatric teams, mostly with too few staff yet with wide responsibilities for cases of many different types. There was a generic approach where teams were responsible for all the problems in their community, which often proved inadequate and problematic. Teams with particular skills and smaller caseloads were formed to provide specialised services, for example assertive outreach, home treatment teams and **early intervention** services with the aim to reduce the need for admission, personality disorder and prison in-reach. **Crisis resolution home treatment (CRHT)** teams helped people through short-term mental health crises by providing intensive treatment and support outside hospital, ideally at home. The National Audit Office reported in December 2007 that the introduction of CRHT teams was associated with reduced pressure on beds, and the teams were successfully reaching service users who would otherwise probably have needed admission (Mays, Dixon and Jones 2011).

The Mental Health Act 1983 was reviewed and *Modernising Mental Health Services* (DoH 1998) proposed a strategy with two essential elements:

- increased investment to provide more beds, outreach facilities and 24-hour access and new treatments; and
- increased control of patients to ensure compliance with treatment in the community, and a new form of revisable detention for those with a severe personality disorder.

In 2001 a White Paper, *Reforming the Mental Health Act*, highlighted the concern that had led to the release of hundreds of patients, some of whom did not receive care, and others becoming a risk to themselves and the community. Such releases had contributed to 1,000 suicides and 40 murders a year from April 1996 to March 2000 (DoH 2001). Finally a new Mental Health Act was passed in 2007, which allowed compulsory treatment in the community under certain circumstances.

Policy, care and treatment for people with mental health problems has been a combination of compassion, fear and control since written records began. Care for people with mental health problems commenced in the community and now is increasingly returning to be a community responsibility. The medicalisation of mental health problems began to be powerful during the increase in asylum provision and is responsible for positive advances in treatments and some awful experiments on people without power by people with power. Today there are still biological, social and psychological explanations of the causes of mental health problems, however these theories are less divided. Research into adverse childhood experiences by Felitti et al. (1998) has influenced the realisation that neglect, abuse and trauma during childhood are influential in the development of many physical and mental health problems in adulthood. There is an increased understanding that positive conditions in early childhood are vital for positive adult mental health. This knowledge, which brings together biological, psychological and social theories, is vital for leading developments in service provision.

This chapter has explored the historical context of mental illness and treatment in terms of biological, social and psychological contexts. Consideration has also been given to how history has helped shape and develop current mental health practices. This includes the influence policy has, which will be explored in more detail in Chapter 3.

REFERENCES

Bartlett (1998) The asylum, the workhouse, and the voice of the insane poor in nineteenth-century England. *International Journal of Law and Psychiatry* 21(4): 421–432.

Beck, A. (1976) *Cognitive therapy and emotional disorders*. New York: New York University Press.

Bentall (2004) *Madness explained: psychosis and human nature*. London: Penguin.

Beresford, P. (2005) Developing self-defined social approaches to madness and distress. In S. Ramon and J. E. Williams (eds), *Mental health at the crossroads: the promise of the psychosocial approach* (pp. 109–123). Aldershot: Ashgate.

Bynum, W. F., Porter, R. and Shepherd, M. (1988) *The anatomy of madness: essays in the history of psychiatry, vol. 3: the asylum and its psychiatry*. London: Routledge.

Carpenter, W. and Davis, J. (2012) Another view of the history of antipsychotic drug discovery and development. *Molecular Psychiatry* 17(12): 1168–1173.

Cherry, S. (2003) *Mental health care in modern England: the Norfolk lunatic asylum.* Suffolk, UK: Boydell Press.

Cummings, I. (2012) Using Simon's *Governing through crime* to explore the development of mental health policy in England and Wales since 1983. *Journal of Social Welfare and Family Law* 34(3): 325–337.

Department of Health (1998) *Modernising mental health services.* London: Department of Health.

Department of Health (2001) *Safety first: five-year report of the national confidential inquiry into suicide and homicide by people with mental illness.* http://webarchive. nationalarchives.gov.uk/20120503230455/http://www.dh.gov.uk/prod_consum_ dh/groups/dh_digitalassets/@dh/@en/documents/digitalasset/dh_4058243.pdf

Descartes, R. (1968) *The philosophical works of Descartes.* Cambridge: Cambridge University Press.

Deutsch, A. (2013) *The mentally ill in America: a history of their care and treatment from colonial times.* Redditch, UK: Read Books.

Felitti, V. J., Anda, R. F. and Nordenberg, D. (1998) Relationship of childhood abuse and household dysfunction to many of the leading causes of death in adults: the adverse childhood experience study. *American Journal of Preventative Medicine* 14: 245–258.

Garrick, M. (2010) Bloodletting 1854: introspection. *American Journal of Psychiatry* 167: 12.

Gibson, M. (2006) *Order from chaos responding to traumatic incidents.* Bristol: Policy Press.

Gilbert, H., Peck, E., Ashton, B., Edwards, N. and Naylor, C. (2014) *Service transformation lessons from mental health.* London: Kings Fund.

Greenstone, G. (2010) The history of bloodletting. *BCMJ* 52(1): 12–14.

Hobert, L. and Binello, E. (2017) Trepanation in Ancient China world. *World Neurosurgery* 101: 451–456.

Howard, S. (2011) *Psychodynamic counselling in a nutshell.* London: Sage.

Islam, F. and Campbell, R. A. (2014) 'Satan has afflicted me!' Jinn-possession and mental illness in the Qur'an. *Journal of Religion and Health* 53(1): 229–243. https:// doi.org/10.1007/s10943-012-9626-5

Kapferer, B. (2003) *Beyond rationalism: Rethinking magic, witchcraft, and sorcery.* New York: Berghahn Books.

Kemp, S. and Williams, K. (1987) Demonic possession and mental disorder in medieval and early modern Europe. *Psychological Medicine* 17(1): 21–29.

The Kings Fund (2014) Service transformation: lessons from mental health. www.kings fund.org.uk/sites/default/files/field/field_publication_file/service-transformation-lessons-mental-health-4-feb-2014.pdf.

Klein, D. and Glick, I. (2014) Industry withdrawal from psychiatric medication development. *Revista Brasileira De Psiquiatria* 36(3): 259–261.

Jacobs, A. (2008) Acid redux: revisiting LSD use in therapy. *Contemporary Justice Review* 11(4): 427–439.

Jones, E. and Wessely, S. (2003) 'Forward psychiatry' in the military: its origins and effectiveness. *Journal of Traumatic Stress* 16(4): 411–419.

Joseph Rowntree Foundation (2018) www.jrf.org.uk/sites/default/files/jrf/migrated/ files/mental-health-service-models-full.pdf

Lidbetter, E. J. (1912) Nature and nurture: a study in conditions. *Eugenics Review* 1: 54–73.

Lloyd, G. (2002) *The man of reason: 'male' and 'female' in Western philosophy.* London: Routledge.

McDonald, A. and Walter, G. (2001) The portrayal of ECT in American movies. *Journal of ECT* 17(4): 264–274.

MacDonald, M. (1981) *Mystical bedlam: madness, anxiety, and healing in seventeenth-century England*. New York: Cambridge University Press.

McKenzie, A. (2012) Anaesthetic and other treatments of shell shock: World War I and beyond. *Journal of the Army Medical Corps* 158(1): 29–33.

Magner, L. N. (1992) *A history of medicine*. New York: Marcel Dekker.

Marston, H. (2013) A brief history of psychiatric drug development. *Journal of Psychopharmacology*. www.bap.org.uk/articles/a-brief-history-of-psychiatric-drug-development

Mays, N., Dixon, A. and Jones, L. (2011) Return to the market: objectives and evolution of New Labour's market reforms. In N. May, A. Dixon and L. Jones (eds), *Understanding New Labour's market reforms of the English NHS* (pp. 1–15). London: The Kings Fund.

Melling, J. (1999) Accommodating madness: new research in the social history of insanity and institutions. In B. Forsythe and J. Melling (eds), *Insanity, institutions and society* (pp. 1–30). New York: Routledge.

National Institute for Health and Care Excellence (NICE) (2005) Clinical guideline [CG26]. Post-traumatic stress disorder: management. www.nice.org.uk/guidance/cg26 (accessed 16 March 2018).

Newnes, C. (2015) *Inscription, diagnosis, deception and the mental health industry: how psy governs us all*. Basingstoke, UK: Macmillan.

Norris, C. (2017) A history of madness: four venerable Virginia lunatic asylums. *Virginia Magazine of History and Biography* 125(2): 138–182.

Pliny, E. M. D. (1854) Bloodletting in mental disorders. *American Journal of Insanity* 10: 293. https://doi.org/10.1176/ajp.10.4.287

Porter, R. (2002) *Madness: a brief history*. New York: Oxford University Press.

Pridmore, S. (2009) *History of psychiatry*. https://eprints.utas.edu.au/287/33/Chapter_28__Electroconvulsive_therapy_(ECT).pdf.pdf (accessed 10 December 2017).

Rae, R. (2007) An historical account of shell shock during the First World War and reforms in mental health in Australia 1914–1939. *International Journal of Mental Health Nursing* 16(4): 266–273.

Rogers, A. and Pilgrim, D. (2001) *Mental health policy in Britain*. Basingstoke, UK: Macmillan Education.

Royal College of Psychiatrists (2013) *The ECT handbook* (3rd ed.). London: Royal College of Psychiatrists.

Sabbatini, R. (1998) The history of shock therapy in psychiatry. *Brain and Mind* 4. www.cerebromente.org.br/n04/historia/shock_i.htm (accessed 10 December 2017).

Scull, A. (1977) *Decarceration: community treatment and the deviant: a radical view* Englewood Cliffs, NJ: Prentice Hall.

Scull, A. (2011) *Madness: a very short introduction*. Oxford: Oxford University Press.

Scull, A. (2014) Some reflections on madness and culture in the post-war world. *History of Psychiatry* 25(4): 395–403. doi: 10.1177/0957154X14546075.

Shryock, R. H. (2006) The psychiatry of Benjamin Rush. *American Journal of Psychiatry* 101(4): 429–432. https://doi.org/10.1176/ajp.101.4.429

Smith, M. (2016) History of mental illness. *Nature* 387: 360.

Spillane, R. (2006) The mind and mental illness: a tale of two myths. *The Skeptic* 26(4): 46–50.

Tatu, L. and Bogousslavsky, J. (2014) World War I psychoneuroses: hysteria goes to war. *Frontiers of Neurology and Neuroscience* 35: 157–168.

Taylor, D. (1984) Understanding the NHS in the 1980s. Office of Health Economics. www.ohe.org/publications/understanding-nhs-1980s

Tyrer and Stienberg (2013) *Models for mental disorder*. Chichester, UK: Wiley Blackwell.

2 MENTAL HEALTH LAW

JO AUGUSTUS AND BRIONY WILLIAMS

INTRODUCTION

Understanding mental health law is essential for all mental health **practitioners**. The Mental Health Act (MHA) 1983 and the Mental Capacity Act (MCA) 2005, along with their associated codes of practice oversee the care and treatment of individuals covered by the definitions in the Acts. In relation to the MCA this relates to all services users and for the MHA this relates to certain service uses (Dimond 2016; Graham and Cowley 2015). This chapter will introduce the MHA and MCA in the context of practice. Although they will not be discussed here, the authors acknowledge that the **Deprivation of Liberty Standards (DoLS)** and the Human Rights Act 1998 also play an important role in mental health law (Department of Health 2005) and their provisions are briefly summarised at the end of the chapter.

BACKGROUND

The purpose of legislation is to set out a framework of rights and responsibilities by which the country is governed. In the UK, the government uses its lawmaking powers to pass legislation in the form of Acts of Parliament. Examples include the Mental Capacity Act 2005 or the **Equality Act 2010**. Sometimes Parliament delegates its lawmaking powers to other government departments, particularly where only a minor change to the law is needed. This is referred to as secondary legislation and leads to the formation of regulations and statutory codes of practice. As an example, in 2012 the coalition government used secondary legislation to amend the list of banned substances contained within the Misuse of Drugs Act 1971, in response to growing concerns about new psychoactive substances (also known as 'legal highs').

In the UK, Parliament has legislative supremacy, meaning that the laws it makes must be followed by the courts (Blakemore and Greene 2004). However, the higher courts still have a role in lawmaking in that the cases they decide shape the interpretation of legislation.

The MCA and MHA were drafted following consultation with key stakeholders including professionals, statutory and voluntary agencies and experts by experience.

Please note that the MCA and MHA are only applicable in England and Wales (not Scotland or Northern Ireland). There are some important amendments to the MHA that are applicable only in Wales and that are outside the scope of this chapter.

WHAT ARE ACTS OF PARLIAMENT, REGULATIONS AND CODES OF PRACTICE?

Acts of Parliament

Acts of Parliament detail the powers, duties, rights and safeguards required by law, where:

- *Powers* may identify what practitioners can lawfully do under the Act. For example, in certain circumstances they may be able to detain someone or otherwise limit their liberty.
- *Duties* specify what these individuals must do in order to exercise such powers.
- *Rights* identify what individuals, e.g. service users, are entitled to. For example, the right to make decisions for themselves wherever it is possible to do so.
- *Safeguards* specify the rights that are in place to protect the individual who is subject to the law. For example, an important safeguard under the MCA is that lack of **capacity** cannot be established 'merely on the basis of a person's age, appearance' or because of 'an aspect of their behaviour which might lead others to make unjustifiable assumptions about their capacity' (MCA 2005, s.3)

In practice, it is essential that the statute balances the mental health professional's powers and duties and safeguards the individual service user.

Regulations

Regulations are secondary legislation (see background above).

Codes of practice

Codes of practice may or may not have statutory effect; they set out further detail that cannot be contained within the primary legislation including, for example, detailed procedures for professionals.

(Dimond 2016; Graham and Cowley 2015; Williamson and Daw 2013)

THE MENTAL CAPACITY ACT 2005

The Mental Capacity Act 2005 (MCA) applies to individuals aged 16 years or older living in England and Wales (although certain sections relate to individuals aged 18 years and over). It provides a legal framework for those who are unable to make all or some decisions for themselves because of an 'impairment of or a disturbance in the functioning of, the brain' (MCA 2005, s.1). For the purposes of the Act, it does not matter whether the impairment or disturbance is permanent or temporary.

Underpinning is the concept that wherever possible, individuals should be allowed to make decisions for themselves or should be assisted to do so. Only where this is not possible should others intervene and make decisions for them. The Act sets out a framework that attempts to enable anyone involved in the provision of care for an individual to assess their capacity (with safeguards). The Act includes a statutory code of practice that must be followed by practitioners.

The MCA took 2 years to implement; it therefore came into force in 2007. It has five key principles. Principles 1, 2 and 3 deal with the establishment of capacity, while principles 4 and 5 deal with decision-making once capacity has been determined. The principles are set out below.

WHAT ARE THE FIVE STATUTORY PRINCIPLES OF THE MCA?

Principle 1

A person must be assumed to have capacity unless it is established that they lack capacity.

Principle 2

A person is not to be treated as unable to make a decision unless all practicable steps to help them to do so have been taken without success.

Principle 3

A person is not to be treated as unable to make a decision merely because they make an unwise decision.

Principle 4

An act done, or decision made, on behalf of a person who lacks capacity, must be done, or made, in their best interests.

Principle 5

Before the act is done, or the decision is made, regard must be had to whether the purpose of the act or the decision can be as effectively achieved in a way that is less restrictive of the person's rights and freedom of action.

(Department of Health 2005)

Lack of capacity may stem from **mental illnesses**, **dementia**, delirium, learning disabilities and some learning difficulties and developmental disabilities such as autism, neurological conditions such as brain injuries or other conditions that cause confusion, drowsiness or loss of consciousness, concussion or coma following an injury, alcohol and drugs (including prescribed treatments) (Department of Health 2005).

To which professionals does the MCA apply?

The MCA applies to all employed professionals who encounter those with issues relating to mental capacity. This includes all health and social care staff from nurses to health care assistants, working in different settings such as voluntary, public and private sector (Williamson and Daw 2013). In addition, the Act applies to friends, family and **carers** of those who lack capacity. Given the kinds of decisions that might have to be made, wider services are also included, such as emergency services and even those providing goods or services such as those working in a bank or building society.

What decisions does the MCA refer to?

The MCA covers most decisions relating to day-to-day activities or needs such as finances, health care or where someone should live.

The provisions of the MCA may apply to hospitals, supported living environments, residential homes, ambulances, police stations or prisons. Decisions covered may include:

- giving **consent** to share information with family and friends, naming specific individuals as requested;
- being admitted to hospital on a voluntary basis as an informal patient;
- consenting to receiving psychiatric treatment;
- making decisions in review meetings of a care plan;
- agreement to receive care, which may be in their own home.

This may include best-interest decisions if the person lacks capacity to consent.

If it becomes apparent that a decision has a higher degree of complexity, then it is important that practitioners seek guidance from the wider team, including perhaps social workers and others. This might be the case where risk of harm to an individual has been identified. It is also important to be aware that there are certain decisions that are not covered by the MCA; primarily this includes decisions covered by the Mental Health Act discussed below (Dimond 2016; Graham and Cowley 2015).

The MCA requires that decisions made under its powers are taken 'on the balance of probabilities'. This means broadly that, given the evidence available, it is more likely than not that an individual lacks capacity. This is a much lower test than is used to establish criminal wrongdoing.

Which decisions are excluded by the MCA?

Certain decisions are excluded from the scope of the MCA, even if the person otherwise lacks capacity. These include:

- consent to have sexual relations;
- consent to marriage or civil partnership;
- consent to divorce or dissolution of civil partnership;
- consent to a child being placed for adoption;
- voting for any decision to be made;
- decisions relating to formal detainment under the MHA.

Practitioners may still be asked to provide their opinion in relation to the above, however, it is important to realise that they are decisions covered by other legislation and so the principles set out in the MCA may not be applicable. Therefore, if decisions relate to the MHA then the MCA should not be applied (Graham and Cowley 2015; Williamson and Daw 2013).

MCA summary

- The MCA deals with the five statutory principles to establish whether someone has capacity to make decisions for themselves and for determining what happens when someone lacks that capacity.
- The MCA supports individuals whenever possible to make their own decisions. This may include people with illness or injury that may find it difficult to make decisions.
- Decisions may include those concerning day-to-day life.
- The MCA primarily applies to those aged 16 years or older and came into force in England and Wales in 2007.
- The MCA can support individuals in planning for the future should they lack capacity to make their own decisions.
- The MCA provides processes to support people to make decisions for those who lack capacity, with safeguards in place (Williamson and Daw 2013).

THE MENTAL HEALTH ACT 1983

The Mental Health Act 1983 (MHA) set out to consolidate all previous laws in relation to 'mentally disordered persons' (MHA 1983, introduction). The Mental Health Act 2007 then amended certain provisions of the MHA 1983 as discussed later in this chapter.

The MHA contains the power to detain and otherwise restrict freedom of 'mentally disordered persons', irrespective of whether or not they have been deemed to have capacity. The MHA provides that a 'mentally disordered person' may be detained for the purposes of assessment, treatment or both, whether it is in their own interest or in the interest of other people.

The MHA has rigid procedures that professionals have to adhere to and safeguards to ensure that the individual is protected, including during aftercare following discharge. The MHA clearly structures the care and treatment for individuals being detained and a code of practice provides more detail. For this reason, the Care Quality Commission (CQC) in England and the Health Inspectorate in Wales inspect all environments where individuals can be detained to ensure procedures and safeguards required under the MHA are in place and have been adhered to (Williamson and Daw 2013; Zigmond and Brindle 2015).

It is fundamental that all mental health professionals have a working knowledge of the MHA, especially those responsible for implementing its specific functions. As part of this there are five sets of overarching principles that must be considered when decisions are being made that relate to the care, support or treatment provision under the MHA. While each principle is of equal importance, there may be variations in their application, depending on the situation. The five principles are as follows (Department of Health 2008):

1. Least restrictive option and maximising independence: Where it is possible to treat a patient safely and lawfully without detaining them under the Act, the patient should not be detained. Wherever possible a patient's independence should be encouraged and supported with a focus on promoting **recovery** wherever possible.
2. **Empowerment** and involvement: Patients should be fully involved in decisions about care, support and treatment. The views of families, carers and others, if appropriate, should be fully considered when taking decisions. Where decisions are taken that are contradictory to views expressed, professionals should explain the reasons for this.
3. Respect and dignity: Patients, their families and carers should be treated with respect and dignity and listened to by professionals.
4. Purpose and effectiveness: Decisions about care and treatment should be appropriate to the patient, with clear therapeutic aims, promote recovery and should be performed to current national guidelines and/or current, available best practice guidelines.
5. Efficiency and equity: Providers, commissioners and other relevant organisations should work together to ensure that the quality of commissioning and provision of mental health care services are of high quality and are given equal priority to physical health and social care services. All relevant services should work together to facilitate timely, safe and supportive discharge from detention.

Family and friends are often an important part of the individual's recovery journey, as Kirsty highlights in Case Study 2.1.

CASE STUDY 2.1: INFORMAL PATIENT EXPERIENCE, KIRSTY'S STORY

In 1986 my husband and I went on holiday to China. I was 3 months' pregnant at the time and I was cleared as fit to travel by my GP. All went well until the penultimate day of the trip. While travelling on the coach I started to bleed heavily (miscarriage). I was then taken by ambulance to hospital and I was operated on. Basically, when I returned home I freaked out. Physically I recovered but mentally I did not. I do not remember exactly when, but I do remember when I was at work I went to the ladies loo screaming and banging on the walls. I also made an unfortunate remark to my husband that I had a thought of drowning myself when I was in the bath. I was diagnosed with an abnormal grief reaction and admitted informally to a mental health hospital.

I recall being sat in a waiting room with a lot of the 'inmates'. Fortunately, a close friend came to be with me and she also brought her young son with her. Eventually I was shown to a room. After she had to leave a care assistant shouted to me, 'Where is your baby gone?', meaning my friend's son, but I didn't take it like that, I was furious and made sure the qualified staff knew what she had done. During my stay I was supremely touched when my younger stepson came to visit me with his dad. However, I had been promised a visit from the minister of the church but he never came. At last I was allowed home and had to return to hospital weekly for follow-ups. I often wanted to scream as the waiting room was shared with the antenatal clinic, just the right environment for me (not).

As Kirsty highlights, a whole-person approach is needed when supporting an individual; this should include spiritual needs as well as practical considerations. All staff should be both aware of and sensitive to the individual's reasons for admission and where possible adjustments made.

MENTAL HEALTH ACT 2007

November 2008 saw the implementation of the MHA 2007, thereby amending certain provisions of the MHA 1983. These amendments included supporting community treatment and reclassifying the types of professionals who can enact detention, under the responsible clinician role (Singh et al. 2017; Williamson and Daw 2013). In addition, the definition of a mental disorder was narrowed from the previous four categories to one category and the distinction previously made between treatable and untreatable conditions (for the purpose of compulsory treatment) was removed. This demonstrated a move towards including those conditions that were previously seen to be untreatable, including those individuals with certain learning disabilities. Arguably, this is a move away from labelling as exclusion, towards inclusivity of individuals towards the provision of assessment and treatment (Singh et al. 2017).

Statutory powers under the MHA summarised (adapted from Department of Health 2008)

Section 2: detention for assessment
Under section 2, a 'patient' may be admitted to hospital and detained for up to 28 days because they are suffering from a 'mental disorder' of a nature or degree that warrants detention and they should be detained because it is in their own interest or in the interest of others.

Section 3: detention for treatment
Under section 3, a 'patient' can be detained in hospital for the purposes of treatment for up to 6 months, however, this can be extended if required. Detention requires an assessment from two doctors.

Section 4: detention in an emergency

Section 4 is used in emergencies only; this is defined in the Act as 'urgent necessity'. A 'patient' can be detained for up to 72 hours, with a recommendation from one doctor, enabling a full assessment to be arranged.

Section 5: holding powers

Section 5 enables certain medical professionals preventing a 'patient' from leaving hospital, if it is believed that it is in their own interest or in the interest of others. Section 5 is only used if it is not possible for sections 2, 3 or 4 to be used. In certain circumstances, nurses may be able to operate limited powers under this section.

   Section 5(2): Doctors' **holding powers**

   Section 5(4): Nurses' holding powers

NB: the individual being detained has the right to challenge their detainment at a tribunal (known as the first-tier tribunal), once in every detainment period.

WHAT ARE NURSE'S HOLDING POWERS?

Consideration to be given during assessment before invoking section 5(4)

Prior to invoking the power, nurses should consider wider factors surrounding the patient. This includes the likely arrival time of the doctor or approved clinician alongside the likely intent of the patient leaving. In addition, consideration must be given to the consequences of the patient leaving the hospital prior to the arrival of the doctor or approved clinician. This includes the risk of harm to self and/or others if the patient were to leave the hospital. The following points need to be considered (Ashmore and Carver 2014):

- the patient's expressed intentions;
- the likelihood of the patient harming themselves or others;
- the likelihood of the patient behaving violently;
- any evidence of disordered thinking;
- the patient's current behaviour and, in particular, any changes in usual behaviour;
- whether the patient has recently received messages from relatives or friends;
- whether the date is one of special significance for the patient – for example, the anniversary of a bereavement;
- any recent disturbances on the ward;
- any relevant involvement of other patients;
- any history of unpredictability or impulsiveness;
- any formal risk assessment that has been undertaken (specifically looking at previous behaviour);
- any other relevant information from other members of the **multidisciplinary team (MDT)**;
- any cases where patients suddenly decide to leave or become determined to do so urgently (Department of Health 2008).

The above box highlights the need for undertaking an ongoing assessment of the patient's needs, in the context of their history and possible risks in the near future. Ashmore and Carver (2000) noted that mental health nurses were seen to be persuading patients to remain in the hospital rather than invoking section 5(4). It is important to note that the code of practice (Department of Health 2008) is seen as encouraging these processes, for example, in the context of waiting until the doctor or approved clinician to arrive. There is, however, a risk of persuasion being viewed as coercive (Ashmore and Carver 2000). Feiring and Ugstad (2014) recognise this as depriving the individual of their liberty and autonomy. This highlights a need for an awareness of persuasion and coercion to be integrated into continuous professional development.

Who is included in an MHA statutory role?

As mentioned previously, the MHA defines specific roles for professionals, family and decision-making groups. These include the following (Williamson and Daw 2013; Zigmond and Brindle 2015):

- An approved clinician is appointed to take responsibility for the treatment of the detained individual. An approved clinician could be a medical doctor, nurse, psychologist, social worker or **occupational therapist**.
- A responsible clinician is an approved clinician allocated to take overall responsibility for the detention of the detained individual. This includes the powers and duties to take leave and discharge, for example. The responsible clinician will review the detained individual ensuring the criteria for detainment is being met.
- An **approved mental health professional (AMHP)** has undertaken specific training and is appointed by the local authority. They are usually a social worker, however, they may also be a nurse, psychologist or occupational therapist. The AMHP applies for the individual to be detained under the MHA.
- The nearest relative is appointed by the AMHP in line with what is listed in the MHA and is given specific responsibilities. This may include a role in the individual's detention or discharge, through provision of information and support.
- **Independent mental health advocates (IMHAs)** are specialist mental health advocates who assist the individual being detained under the Mental Health Act, or those who are subject to its powers under **community treatment orders** or guardianship.
- Second-opinion approved doctor (SOAD) is a psychiatrist appointed by the CQC to provide another opinion on medical treatment for an individual detained under the MHA.

MHA summary

- An individual can only be detained if they have a mental health disorder and meet the criteria for detention.
- An initial detention under the MHA is recommended by medical practitioners and can be renewed by two professionals.
- An individual can be detained for up to 72 hours in an emergency, up to 28 days for assessment and up to 6 months for treatment. This must be under constant review to ensure that criteria are being met.
- The individual being detained may challenge their detention at the tribunal.
- Advocacy must be made available to the individual being detained.
- There are emergency provisions under the Act that may be applied to allow short-term detention.

HUMAN RIGHTS ACT 1998

The Human Rights Act 1998 incorporated into UK law certain rights and freedoms set out in the European Convention on Human Rights (these are known as the Convention Rights). The Act sets out people's rights in a series of 'Articles', for example, Article 5 is the right to liberty and security and Article 8 is the right to respect for private and family life, home and correspondence.

The Act makes it unlawful for any public authority to act in a way that is inconsistent with Convention Rights and requires the judiciary to interpret legislation in a way that is consistent with them. The Conservative government under David Cameron proposed repeal of the Human Rights Act, replacing it instead with a 'British Bill of Rights'.

DEPRIVATION OF LIBERTY SAFEGUARDS (DOLS)

The Deprivation of Liberty Safeguards amended the Mental Capacity Act 2005 to provide certain safeguards where restraint is used to deprive someone of their liberty within a care home or hospital setting. A series of assessments must be undertaken to determine whether someone's liberty can be deprived. The safeguards include, for example, provision for someone to be represented and for them to be afforded a right of appeal against detention.

This chapter has considered the key components of both mental health law and policy. Detail has been provided about the Mental Health Act (MHA) 1983 and the Mental Capacity Act (MCA) 2005, along with their associated codes of practice to oversee the care and treatment of individuals covered be the definitions in the Acts. In addition, an overview of the Deprivation of Liberty Standards (DoLS) and the Human Rights Act 1998 is given, as they play an important role in mental health law. Consideration has also been given to policy and the role it has at both a local and national level. While the **mental health** priorities outlined in this chapter are current at the time of writing, it is important to acknowledge that these are subject to change. However, they remain relevant as new policies are often developed from historic policy. There is a recognition that all mental health professionals need to hold a working knowledge of what law and policy means for the individual, their family and/or carers. Such competence will support the delivery of **person-centred care** and in turn promote recovery.

REFERENCES

Ashmore, R. and Carver, N. (2000) De facto detentions: why mental health nurses may be avoiding using section 5(4). *Mental Health Practice* 3(5): 12–18.

Ashmore, R. and Carver, N. (2014) Understanding and implementing the nurse's holding power (section 5(4)) of the Mental Health Act 1983. *Mental Health Practice* 18(1): 30–36.

Blakemore, T. and Greene, B. (2004) *Law for legal executives*. Oxford: Oxford University Press.

Department of Health (2005) *Mental Capacity Act*. London: HMSO.

Department of Health (2008) *Code of practice: Mental Health Act 1983.* London: HMSO.

Dimond, B. (2016) *Legal aspects of mental capacity: a practical guide for health and social care professionals.* London: Wiley-Blackwell.

Graham, M. and Cowley, J. (2015) *A practical guide to the Mental Capacity Act 2005: putting the principles of the act into practice.* London: Jessica Kingsley Publishers.

Feiring, E. and Ugstad, K. (2014) Interpretations of legal criteria for involuntary psychiatric admission: a qualitative analysis. *BMC Health Services Research* 14(1): 500–509.

Human Rights Act (1998) c42. www.legislation.gov.uk/ukpga/1998/42 (accessed 16 February 2017).

Mental Capacity Act (2005) c9. www.legislation.gov.uk/ukpga/2005/9/contents (accessed 16 February 2017).

Mental Health Act (1983) c.20. www.legislation.gov.uk/ukpga/1983/20/contents (accessed 16 May 2018).

Mental Health Act (2007) c12. www.legislation.gov.uk/ukpga/2007/12/contents (accessed 16 February 2017).

Singh, S., Paul, M., Parsons, H., Burns, T., Tyrer, P., Fazel, S., Deb, S., Islam, Z., Rugkåsa, J., Gajwani, R., Thana, L. and Crawford, M. (2017) A prospective, quantitative study of mental health act assessments in England following the 2007 amendments to the 1983 act: did the changes fulfill their promise? *BMC Psychiatry* 17: 1–8.

Williamson, T. and Daw, R. (2013) *Law, values and practice in mental health nursing: a handbook.* Maidenhead, UK: Open University Press.

Zigmond, T. and Brindle, N. (2015) *A clinician's brief guide to the Mental Health Act.* London: Royal College of Psychiatrists.

3 MENTAL HEALTH POLICY

JO AUGUSTUS AND BRIONY WILLIAMS

LEARNING OBJECTIVES

After studying this chapter you will be able to:

- understand the context of mental health policy at a national and local level;
- describe the current **mental health** priorities;
- understand the factors that influence policy;
- explore examples of serious case reviews.

INTRODUCTION

A policy is a plan of action that affects what we do and how we do it. It is a statement of intent and contains basic principles to guide practice. A good policy also contains achievable objectives implemented as a procedure or protocol. Rogers and Pilgrim (2001, p. 226) state that any policy should be involved with:

- legal arrangements;
- service investments;
- control of behaviour.

Sealey (2015) explains that a policy occurs from an identified need or issue and is usually but not always made by consultation between interested parties. A policy has a specific aim, criteria for success in order to measure if it has been effective, and is usually made by those in power. Policy can be national, international, local and within organisations. International and national policy shapes legislation and provides the context in which legislation should be viewed. It also alerts us to what is coming next. Local and organisational policies are about how the legislation will be implemented in those particular settings.

POLICY AND LEGISLATION

The term legislation means statutory law and is the legal framework in which any policy exists. Legislation is also the process of making law. There are many different types of national and local policy, which inform strategies that affect mental health services, but all policies have to be written with the consideration of legislation.

An example of a local organisational policy

Dealing with harassment and bullying policy.

Purpose

Outlines the purpose of the policy and links with the Equality Act and the local policy of equality and diversity. Discusses the organisational commitment to an environment where people are treated with dignity and respect.

Overview

Discusses the reasons why this policy is important and the impact of bullying and harassment on people. Explains the key themes and the effects on the organisation. Sets out the disciplinary penalties for people who engage in bullying and harassment.

Scope

Gives examples of bullying and harassment.

Outline of the policy

Mentions all the people who are covered by the policy and different types of bullying and harassment.

Sets out a set of behaviours for the following groups:

- the organisation;
- staff and users of the organisation;
- management; and
- advisors.

How a national policy is made

Before a general election, each political party sets out their ideas and plans regarding policy changes they aim to make if they get into power, related to the issues they believe are important. The public ideally listen to the aims and changes suggested, and vote for the political party with the most policies that they agree with. However, post-election some proposed policy plans/changes do not ever become policy or they get changed in the process of discussion and formulation. The policies that become implemented, and how quickly, depend on a number of factors. For example, if a government has a strong majority, the policies may follow from their reaction to a number of high-profile media events. Policy change in the past has not always been evidence based and has sometimes been a reaction to a high-profile event. It can be difficult to reach a compromise and satisfy all the views of interested parties, for example staff working in mental health services, service users, **carers** and action groups may have different opinions on the priorities and the way forward. Government ministers have been criticised for not prioritising mental health in their general health policy.

MENTAL HEALTH POLICY

Mental health policy sets out the vision for the future mental health of the population, stating the framework that will be put in place to manage and prevent priority mental and neurological disorders (WHO 2017). According to Rogers and Pigrim (2001, p. 226), mental health policy is concerned with promoting well-being, ameliorating distress and controlling behaviour. Another way of expressing this is that it is about prevention, reducing distress and compulsion. Therefore, it is:

- responding to current identified mental health issues;
- creating plans to prevent potential future mental health problems;
- setting up services to help improve the lives of people who have mental health problems;
- creating rules to safeguard people with mental health problems and the wider public.

Any mental health policy should include concrete strategies and actions that will be implemented to tackle mental health problems, as well as specifying the targets to be achieved by the government both nationally and locally. It should also clarify the roles of different stakeholders in implementing the actions of the mental health policy (WHO 2017). One of the factors that may impact on the process could be the **stigma** around mental health. Jenkins (2003) proposes that in developing mental health policy, it is important to include consideration of stigma about mental health issues and **mental illness**. Jenkins (2003) says stigma creates a lack of attention from ministers and the public, which then results in a lack of resource and morale, decaying institutions, lack of leadership, inadequate information systems and inadequate legislation. NHS England published its commissioned Mental Health Taskforce report in 2016, including its *Five Year Forward View for Mental Health* and *Implementation Plan* (NHS England 2016b). Although prevention was highlighted as a key priority by the public engagement exercise carried out beforehand, the final taskforce recommendations were not as strong on prevention as was hoped. The box below summarises the key mental health polices and strategies in the UK.

Points to consider

UK government policies and strategies specific to mental health:

- 1999 National Service Framework for Adult Mental Health Services
- 2000 The NHS Plan
- 2004 National Service Framework for Children, Young People and Maternity Services
- 2005 Delivering Race Equality
- 2007 Improving Access to Psychological Therapies (IAPT)
- 2009 The Bradley Report
- 2011 No Health Without Mental Health
- 2014 Crisis Care Concordat
- 2016 Five Year Forward View
- 2017 Mental Health Service Reform.

Who informs the government?

Health and care professionals

Staff who work in mental health services such as psychiatrists, clinical psychologists, mental health or child nurses, social workers and **occupational therapists** are represented by a professional body who are independent from the government, for example the Royal College of Psychiatrists, Royal College of Nursing and the Royal College of Occupational Therapists. Each professional body canvasses staff and produces reports for policy makers on relevant topics. Some professions are linked through their regulatory body such as the Health and Care Professions Council. Staff are also represented through the management structure in the NHS, social care or public health. Each staff group has a different viewpoint, for example psychiatrists may have a more medical model understanding of mental health and the priorities and the direction that needs to be taken, whereas clinical psychologists and social workers may have a more psychological or social view of the shape of services. There are also wider groups of staff who have an interest in mental health and influence policy changes, such as probation officers and people working in the court system, youth workers, clergy and teachers. They make their views known through pressure groups and through their professional body.

Advisory bodies

Advisory bodies and watchdogs such as the Care Quality Commission (CQC) and the National Institute for Health and Care Excellence (NICE) are independent and not controlled by central government. They are known as quasi-autonomous, non-governmental organisations (quangos). The Equality and Human Rights Council (EHRC) (2017) states that it is

> a statutory non-departmental public body established by the Equality Act 2006, the Commission operates independently. We aim to be an expert and authoritative organisation that is a centre of excellence for evidence, analysis and equality and human rights law. We also aspire to be an essential point of contact for policy makers, public bodies and business.

Quangos are funded by taxpayers, therefore it could be argued how independent from government they can be. Cavadino (1995) states that governments can protect themselves from criticism by hiding behind bodies that project themselves as independent but are in reality government controlled, thus exerting power without responsibility. For example, the Mental Health Act Commission (MHAC) was set up in 1983 and was allowed and encouraged to act as if it were independent, but ultimately, as Cavadino (1995) argues, 'it was on the end of a long rope that could always be hauled in if it was thought to be necessary' (p. 57). The MHAC has now been replaced by the CQC, which monitors, inspects and regulates services to make sure they meet fundamental standards of quality and safety and publishes what it finds, including performance ratings to help people choose care. Many quangos were created by the Labour government and then axed by the coalition and Conservative governments as part of the Health and Care Act (2012) as they were very expensive to run. Some of their work was absorbed by central government or taken on by charities and the **voluntary sector**.

Service users and carers

Service users and carers inform and campaign for policy change either through their own initiative or through charity organisations such as Rethink and Mind, mental health charities who provide support and advice and campaign to change policy and improve services. All general public are service users and carers and thus individuals can campaign for change by gathering signatures on the government website and this then has to be discussed in Parliament.

The Mental Health Taskforce chaired by Mind chief executive Paul Farmer in 2016 brought together health and care leaders, service users and mental health experts to create a 5-year plan for mental health care in England. The Mental Health Task Force worked closely with organisations including NHS England and Rethink Mental Illness to ensure their voices were heard. Other organisations that work to influence mental health policy include:

- The Joseph Rowntree Foundation: an independent organisation working to inspire social change through research, policy and practice.
- The Centre for Mental Health (previously known as the Sainsbury Centre for Mental Health): influential in the development of the National Service Frameworks in Mental Health (1999), it is now an entirely independent charity, working to create a fairer chance in life for people with mental health problems through life-changing research.

The Centre for Mental Health aims to change the lives of people with mental health problems by using research to bring about better services and fairer policies.

- The Mental Health Foundation: a charity with prevention at the heart of what it does and that aims to find and address the sources of mental health problems.

HISTORY OF POLICY

The history of mental health policy and services shows us how governments build on, remove or change policy over time. As discussed in Chapter 1, people with mental health problems were historically cared for by their family and community. In the 1700s institutions were set up to look after and segregate those with mental health problems. The last 100 years of mental health policy has seen a decline of the large institutions and an increase of treatment and support in the community. This was in part due to the developments in pharmacology and the invention of major tranquilisers, which made it easier to treat people with psychosis. Another factor is an increased recognition of human rights. However, the change was most likely due to the cost of looking after the numbers of people who were admitted for treatment and the realisation that many people did not need inpatient care.

The move of services into the community took place over a few decades and was not without its critiques. The National Service Framework in Mental Health (NSF) (1999) was a significant change in how community services were organised. Previously all community services were through **community mental health teams** after the NSF specialist teams were formed to concentrate on specific aspects of provision. Crisis teams, assertive outreach teams and **early intervention** for psychosis teams were set up containing staff with specialist knowledge. The National Institute of Clinical Excellence (NICE) was set up to ensure treatments and service changes were **evidence based**. 'At a national level, official health and social care research and development programmes are now in place and actively commissioning research to provide [an] underpinning evidence base for policy and practice' (Lester and Glasby 2010, p. 19).

MENTAL HEALTH POLICY UNDER THE 2015 GOVERNMENT

Under the coalition government from 2010 to 2015, the mental health service reform government policy was implemented (DoH 2016b). This identified poor mental health as the largest cause of disability in the UK, in conjunction with social problems such as education and poor physical health. This highlighted the importance of improving an individual's mental health and well-being in order to improve all other areas of life. In response to this various campaigns and initiatives were launched, including:

- improving access to psychological therapies service provision;
- the Time to Change campaign to reduce stigma surrounding mental health;
- preventing suicides and improving mental health service provision for veterans.

Although improving public health, modernising **primary care** and mental health provision for older people and children were core standards in the National Service Frameworks, limited progress was made in these areas (Kings Fund 2014). The concept of the 'big society', whereby citizens would take more control over their lives and build more capable communities, was put forward by the coalition government. National policy has become more supportive of local innovation, with an increasing emphasis on broadening access to mental health services beyond those with severe mental illness. One of the most influential recent policies has been the Improving Access to Psychological Therapies (IAPT) programme, which was established in 2006 and allocated funding of £33 million in the first year and £70 million each year for a further 2 years under the 2007 comprehensive spending review (Kings Fund 2014). The Mental Health Policy Group, consisting of the Centre for Mental Health, Mental Health Foundation, Mental Health Network, Mind, Rethink Mental Illness and the Royal College of Psychiatrists, joined forces to produce a plan for what the government must do in the first 100 days of the new Parliament in order to improve the lives of people with mental health problems. The 2016 plan sets out a number of practical actions the government should take to ensure mental and physical health are valued equally. Liberal Democrat MP Norman Lamb is both a mental health campaigner and a member of Parliament; he was health minister in the coalition government. He has a personal motivation for wanting change as both his son and his sister have suffered from mental health problems. This personal rationale for an MP may benefit the development of mental health policy and funding for change by keeping mental health in the media and ensuring it remains a priority for action.

CURRENT MENTAL HEALTH PRIORITIES

The 'big society' concept of the coalition government changed under the Conservative government who were elected in 2015 and became instead the 'shared society', as named by Prime Minister Theresa May. A 'shared society' is where we all have responsibilities to and for each other, including businesses and charities. The government has a responsibility to step in to help the following priorities:

- identification and treatment of **anxiety** and **depression** for women during pregnancy and after childbirth;
- treatment of conduct disorder in young children;
- early intervention services for first-episode psychosis;
- liaison psychiatry services in acute hospitals;
- integrated care for people with long-term physical and mental health conditions;
- improved management of medically unexplained symptoms and related complex needs;
- supported employment services for people with severe mental illness;
- community-based alternatives to acute inpatient care for people in a crisis;
- interventions to improve the physical health of people with severe mental illness, especially smoking cessation.

WHAT FACTORS INFLUENCE MENTAL HEALTH POLICY?

Cost economics

The introduction of antipsychotic drugs and mood stabilisers allowed more people to be treated in the community, and outpatient clinic attendances increased from virtually zero in 1930 to 144,000 in 1959 (Lester and Glasby 2010).

The Centre for Mental Health (2016) states that the economic and social costs of mental health problems in England in 2009/10 was £105.2 billion. This figure includes:

- costs of health and social care for people with mental health problems;
- lost output in the economy from sickness absence and unemployment;
- human costs of reduced quality of life.

The *Five Year Forward View for Mental Health* (NHS England 2016b) made a set of recommendations to put mental health on a par with physical health to achieve the ambition of parity of esteem. A 2016 policy document, 'Improving the Physical Health of People with Mental Health Problems: Actions for Mental Health Nurses', from the Nursing, Midwifery and Allied Health Professions Policy Unit, states:

> People with severe mental illness are particularly at risk and die on average 15–20 years earlier than the general population. Being in contact with mental health services does not necessarily mean that people will have a physical health assessment, have their physical health monitored, or receive the information and support they need to adopt a healthier lifestyle. (DoH 2016a, p. 1)

One of the reasons that parity of esteem is a priority is due to the high cost of hospital treatment that could be preventable. NHS England has agreed that by 2020/1 at least 280,000 more people living with severe mental health problems should have their physical health needs met. One of the ways that this can be achieved is through the Commissioning for Quality and Innovation (CQUIN) payment framework. This enables commissioners of services to reward excellence among providers of mental health services through the achievement of quality improvement goals (NHS England 2016a).

Increased services for women with perinatal mental health problems are in part informed by the economic and social long-term cost to society of about £8.1 billion for each 1-year cohort of births in the UK. Perinatal mental health problems affect up to 20% of women at some point during the perinatal period. They are also of major importance as a public health issue, not just because of their adverse impact on the mother but also because they have been shown to compromise the healthy emotional, cognitive and even physical development of the child, with serious long-term consequences (Bauer et al. 2014).

MEDIA ATTENTION

Media influences public attitudes towards mental illness and policy development. The policy of community care for people with mental illness came under intense scrutiny during the 1990s, following a series of homicides and incidents of violence, suicide and neglect involving people with mental health problems. The media appeared to be particularly successful in highlighting such cases, influencing public opinion and inspiring policy responses (Hallam 2002). The high-profile case of Christopher Clunis, who had a diagnosis of **schizophrenia** and murdered Jonathan Zito in an unprovoked attack, highlighted the potential consequences of community patients losing contact with mental health services. This resulted in a growing policy focus on people with severe mental illness and risk management, public safety and containment.

The implementation of the **Care Programme Approach (CPA)** in 1990, which is still a fundamental framework within which mental health services operate, attempted to improve continuity of care for people with mental health problems. Cummins (2012) argues that the media coverage of high-profile cases led to the introduction of increasingly restrictive and bureaucratic approaches.

SERIOUS CASE REVIEWS

Winterbourne View
Winterbourne View was an independent inpatient hospital that opened in 2006 in the North Bristol area to provide assessment, treatment and rehabilitation for individuals with learning disabilities. It was closed on 31 May 2011 after a media investigation brought to light acts of criminal activity that were being conducted by staff. Different investigations then took place including the following:

- A serious case review, conducted by South Gloucestershire Safeguarding Adults Board.
- The police launched investigations that led to 11 criminal convictions.
- The Care Quality Commission (CQC) inspected all health care settings operated by the owners of Winterbourne View. They also then inspected all learning disability **service providers** in England.

Mid Staffordshire NHS Foundation Trust Public Inquiry
In 2008 the Healthcare Commission highlighted high numbers of patient deaths in Mid Staffordshire NHS Foundation Trust that were linked to poor standards of care. Subsequently, in 2009 Robert Francis QC began an investigation. In 2013 the final Francis Report was published, identifying serious failings in care between 2005 and 2008, which included neglect and abuse that in some instances led to avoidable deaths. The report identified appalling standards of care, linked to the development of poor standards within the culture of the organisation over a period of time. For example, staff being driven by tasks rather than prioritising patient-centred care. As a consequence of the Francis Report, recommendations were made specifically to NHS staff with regard to duty of openness, transparency and candour.

WHAT IS A SERIOUS CASE REVIEW, A SAFEGUARDING ADULTS BOARD AND DUTY OF CANDOUR?

Serious case review

A serious case review is a process for all agencies and is often triggered when serious and/or complex safeguarding issues are highlighted in care practice, such as at Winterborne View. More specifically, where incidences of abuse of neglect are suspected or if a vulnerable adult has died or been seriously injured. It is seen as a shift away from a blame culture, instead focusing on lessons learnt in order to improve care practices.

Safeguarding Adults Board (SAB)

The SAB is in place to safeguard adults who have care and support needs and who may be identified as vulnerable adults. This is done by ensuring local safeguarding arrangements are in place, as stated in the Care Act 2014 and also ensuring that safeguarding arrangements are patient centred and focused on positive outcomes. To facilitate this, agencies need to work collaboratively to prevent abuse and neglect and ensure a continuous cycle of improvement happens in the reporting processes.

Duty of candour

Duty of candour is a statutory or legal requirement to be open and honest, when something goes wrong and may have caused or could cause serious harm. This is referred to in the Francis Report in terms of openness, transparency and candour for all health and care providers registered with the Care Quality Commission.

Impact of generic policy

The Health and Social Care Act (2012) is an Act of Parliament made during the coalition government. It sets out the reorganisation of the structure of the NHS in England. 'The Health and Social Care Act (2012) puts clinicians at the centre of commissioning, frees up providers to innovate, empowers patients and gives a new focus to public health' (Department of Health 2012). As part of the Act, Public Health England was established as an executive agency of the Department of Health, working at a local level, driving health improvement on issues such as mental illness, disability and harm from alcohol, drugs and smoking. The **Equality Act (2010)** brings together many pieces of legislation into one single Act. The Act provides a legal framework to protect the rights of individuals and advance equality of opportunity for all. Mental impairment is one of the protected characteristics in the disability section of the Act, which aims to protect individuals with mental health problems from unfair treatment. Table 3.2 sets out the key legislation and policy that currently affects mental health services.

Table 3.2 Key legislation and policy affecting mental health services

Government	Year	Policy
Labour	1999	National Service Framework for Mental Health was launched to establish a comprehensive evidence-based service
	2000	NHS Plan set targets and provided funding to make the Framework a reality
	2004	National Service Framework for Children, Young People and Maternity Services
	2007	Reform of the Mental Health Act
Coalition	2011	Mental health strategy set six objectives, including improvement in the outcomes, physical health and experience of care of people with mental health problems, and a reduction in avoidable harm and stigma
	2011	No Health Without Mental Health
Conservative	2015	Future in Mind
		Consensus about the way in which it can be made easier for children and young people to access high-quality mental health care when they need it
	2016	Five Year Forward View

REFERENCES

Bauer, A., Parsonage, M., Knapp, M., Iemmi, V. and Adelaja, B. (2014) *Costs of perinatal mental health problems*. London: LSE and Centre for Mental Health.

Cavadino, M. (1995) Quasi-government: the case of the Mental Health Act Commission. *International Journal of Public Sector Management* 8(7): 56–62. http://dx.doi.org/10.1108/09513559510103184.

Centre for Mental Health (2016) https://www.centreformentalhealth.org.uk/publications/implementing-mental-health-policy-some-lessons-recent-history-0.

Cummins, I. (2012) Using Simon's *Governing through crime* to explore the development of mental health policy in England and Wales since 1983. *Journal of Social Welfare and Family Law* 34(3): 325–337.

Department of Health (2011) No health without mental health: a cross-government mental health outcomes strategy for people of all ages. www.gov.uk/government/publications/the-mental-health-strategy-for-england.

Department of Health (2016a) Improving the physical health of people with mental health problems: actions for mental health nurses. https://assets.publishing.service.gov.uk/government/uploads/system/uploads/attachment_data/file/532253/JRA_Physical_Health_revised.pdf.

Department of Health (2016b) Mental health service reform. www.gov.uk/government/policies/mental-health-service-reform.

Department of Health and Care Act (2012) https://services.parliament.uk/bills/2010-11/healthandsocialcare.html.

The Equality Act (2010) www.legislation.gov.uk/ukpga/2010/15/contents.

Equality and Human Rights Council (EHRC) (2017) www.equalityhumanrights.com/en/about-us/who-we-are.

Hallam, A. (2002) Media influences on mental health policy: long-term effects of the Clunis and Silcock cases. *International Review of Psychiatry* 14(1): 26–33.

Jenkins, R. (2003) Supporting governments to adopt mental health policies. *World Psychiatry* 2(1): 14–19.

The Kings Fund (2014) www.kingsfund.org.uk/sites/files/kf/field/field_publication_file/service-transformation-lessons-mental-health-4-feb-2014.pdf.

Lester, H. and Glasby, J. (2010) *Mental health policy and practice* (2nd ed.). Basingstoke, UK: Palgrave Macmillan.

NHS England (2016a) Commissioning for quality and innovation (CQUIN) guidance for 2015/16. March. www.england.nhs.uk/nhs-standard-contract/cquin/cquin-16-17.

NHS England (2016b) Mental Health Taskforce report: Five Year Forward View and Implementation Plan. www.england.nhs.uk/mental-health/taskforce.

Rogers, A. and Pilgrim, D. (2001) *Mental health policy in Britain* (2nd ed.). London: Palgrave Macmillan.

Sealey, C. (2015) *Social policy simplified connecting theory with people's lives*. London: Palgrave Macmillan.

Time To Change (2017) Mind and rethink mental illness. www.time-to-change.org.uk.

World Health Organisation (2017) *Mental health policy and service development*. Geneva: WHO, Department of Mental Health and Substance Abuse. www.who.int/mental_health/policy/services/en.

4 MENTAL HEALTH PROFESSIONALS

JO AUGUSTUS AND JUSTINE BOLD

LEARNING OBJECTIVES

After studying this chapter you will be able to:

- understand the background to the provision of mental health services;
- describe the mental health professionals who may be involved in an individual's care;
- understand the regulatory bodies that mental health professionals may be registered with;
- consider the different types of **service providers**.

Mental health service provision offers evidence-based interventions for a variety of different conditions that impact on an individual's **psychological well-being**. This can be undertaken in a variety of different settings and across the individual's life course (WHO 2008). Before detailing the different professions that work in mental health services, the chapter will consider how services are commissioned, as well as exploring the different types of services.

Clinical Commissioning Groups (CCG) largely commission mental health services for their local communities. CCGs were formed following the introduction of the Health and Social Care Act in 2012, replacing the Primary Care Trusts. To date there are 209 CCGs in England (Hayden 2011).

WHAT IS COMMISSIONING?

Commissioning focuses on getting the best possible health outcomes for the local community. This is done by assessing local needs and then buying services on behalf of the population from service providers, e.g. hospitals. This is an ongoing process where CCGs must respond to an ever-changing local community and their success is measured by improvement in patient outcomes, such as a reduction in symptoms.

- CCGs are run by an elected governing body, which is made up of a variety of clinicians, such as GPs, nurses, **consultants** and other lay members.
- CCGs hold responsibility for two-thirds of the total NHS budget, which is £71.9 billion for 2016/17.
- Although CCGs are independent, they are accountable to the Secretary of State for Health.

(Coleman et al. 2015)

Mental health services are provided by different organisational bodies including the NHS, private sector, charities and social enterprises. Such services are primarily accessed by a GP referral, although some accept self-referrals, e.g. Improving Access to Psychological Therapies (IAPT). The waiting time for accessing services across England varies, although organisations can be subject to penalties if targets are not reached (Williams 2015). In order to meet the required target and meet the needs of the clinical population, mental health providers are required to employ a variety of professional staff and settings (Richards and Borglin 2011). Such professions may be regulated by professional bodies, although many are unregulated. However, Skills for Care developed the Care Certificate, which outlines the minimum standards a health care professional should develop when embarking on their career (Ashurst 2015). Although this is not a form of professional regulation, the Care Certificate bridges the gap between professional and non-professional workforce. In other words, the difference between individuals that have undertaken academic training, often at postgraduate level, which is regulated by a professional body.

WHO ARE THE REGULATORY BODIES, WHO REGULATES WHO?

British Association for Counselling and Psychotherapy (BACP)

Supports the practice of the counselling professions, including psychotherapists to improve psychological well-being and **mental health**, while promoting social justice in the context of diverse community settings.

Roles include: psychotherapists, counsellors, genetic counsellors, humanistic, psychodynamic, transactional analysis, Gestalt, psychoanalytical, family therapy.

British Association for Behavioural and Cognitive Psychotherapies (BABCP)

Provides a multidisciplinary platform for those practising in the theory and practice of cognitive and behavioural psychotherapies.

Roles include: cognitive behavioural therapists.

(Continued)

(Continued)

Royal College of Psychiatrists

Aspires to improve the outcomes of individuals with mental health difficulties, as well as their families and the surrounding community.

Roles include: psychiatrists.

General Medical Council (GMC)

Facilitates the protection of service users and develops medical education as well as clinical practice.

Roles include: doctors.

Health and Care Professions Council (HCPC)

Established to protect the public by holding a register of health and care professionals who meet the required training competencies.

Roles include: arts therapists, biomedical scientists, chiropodists/podiatrists, clinical scientists, dieticians, hearing aid dispensers, **occupational therapists**, operating department **practitioners**, orthoptists, paramedics, physiotherapists, practitioner psychologists, prosthetists/orthotists, radiographers, social workers in England and speech and language therapists.

Nursing and Midwifery Council (NMC)

Provides a standard of education enabling nurses and midwives to provide a high standard of health care provision, which also includes conduct.

Roles include: child and adolescent mental health nurses, adult mental health nurses, community mental health nurses, adult and children's nursing and midwifery.

The type of mental health service accessed depends on a variety of factors, such as the individual's age, the severity of their problem and their diagnosis. The National Institute for Health and Care Excellence (NICE) recommends a stepped model of care that denotes a variety of evidence-based psychological interventions to promote **recovery** (Ekers and Webster 2012). It is based on the following two principles:

1. The most effective and least intrusive intervention should be offered in the first instance.
2. An individual's progress should be regularly reviewed to establish if their needs are met at the same or a different step.

The stepped-care model provides a framework in which to organise the provision of services, and supports patients, **carers** and practitioners in identifying and accessing the most effective interventions (see Table 4.1). In stepped care the least intrusive,

Table 4.1 Stepped-care model

Focus of the intervention	Nature of the intervention
STEP 4: Severe and complex[a] depression, risk to life, severe self-neglect	Medication, high-intensity psychological interventions, electroconvulsive therapy, crisis service, combined treatments, multiprofessional and inpatient care
STEP 3: Persistent subthreshold depressive symptoms or mild to moderate depression with inadequate response to initial interventions, moderate and severe depression	Medication, high-intensity psychological interventions, combined treatments, collaborative care[b] and referral for further assessment and interventions
STEP 2: Persistent subthreshold depressive symptoms, mild to moderate depression	Low-intensity psychosocial interventions, psychological interventions, medication and referral for further assessment and interventions
STEP 1: All known and suspected presentations of depression	Assessment, support, psychoeducation, active monitoring and referral for further assessment and interventions

[a] Complex depression includes depression that shows an inadequate response to multiple treatments, is complicated by psychotic symptoms, and/or is associated with significant psychiatric comorbidity or psychosocial factors.

[b] Only for depression where the person also has a chronic physical health problem and associated functional impairment (see depression in adults with a chronic physical health problem: recognition and management [NICE clinical guideline 91]).

Source: Reproduced with permission under the terms of the NICE UK Open Content Licence.

most effective intervention is provided first; if a person does not benefit from the intervention initially offered, or declines an intervention, they should be offered an appropriate intervention from the next step.

The stepped-care model is used to manage the provision of psychological therapies and also to enable choice for individuals, their family and carers. The model provides an overview of an integrated pathway for both assessment and treatment of common mental health problems, as well as more complex presentations (National Institute for Health and Clinical Excellence 2011; Richards et al. 2012). The commissioning of such stepped-care services is likely to be cost effective, produce better patient outcomes and greater patient satisfaction. This is as a result of the least intensive outcome limiting the disease burden and costs incurred in more intensive interventions. It is also expected that if symptom relief is gained at the first intervention used and choice is given, then the patient's experience is likely to be positive (Ekers and Webster 2012). This approach offers flexibility, as service users can start treatment at any stage of the stepped-care model. However, it is also important to note that service provision does vary geographically and therefore there may be some restrictions in place. For example, service users may have to start engaging at steps 1–3 before being referred to secondary services, as Case Study 4.1 explores.

CASE STUDY 4.1: A DIAGNOSIS OF SCHIZOPHRENIA, ROD'S STORY

Rod was diagnosed with **schizophrenia** in his late twenties, after being admitted to hospital under the Mental Health Act, on six different occasions. Now, 10 years later he has been living in a supported community and his symptoms stabilised enough for him to be working 10 hours a week. Six months ago Rod's GP diagnosed and treated him for shingles; it took around 2 months for him to recover fully. During these 2 months Rod increasingly became isolated and began to have panic attacks when he had to leave his flat. His support workers became increasingly concerned about Rod's deteriorating mental health and referred him to his psychiatrist, with a view to receiving treatment from **secondary care**. However, following the psychiatric assessment, his psychiatrist recommended he engage in face-to-face **cognitive behaviour therapy (CBT)** to overcome symptoms of **panic disorder** with agoraphobia supported by his support workers.

Question: Given his diagnosis of schizophrenia, which he has been previously treated for in secondary care services, why might Rod be referred for CBT **primary care** service provision?

Hint: Refer back to the two guiding principles of the stepped-care model.

Therefore, if the stepped-care model is applied in a patient-centred way, consistently between mental health professionals, it can promote recovery. Indeed, referral to a higher or lower step of the model may also save money and incur a shorter waiting time. Research into the effectiveness of the stepped model and its provision in services concluded that there have been both improved patient outcomes and recovery rates (NHS Confederation 2011). However, such effective outcomes are reliant on staff following NICE guidance and for this to happen services have to be available (Von Korff and Goldberg 2001). Thus, staff need to be trained in NICE guidance and such knowledge needs to be kept up to date, which is both the responsibility of the individual employee and employer.

WHERE DO MENTAL HEALTH PROFESSIONALS WORK?

It is possible for anyone with an interest in working in mental health to gain a position in a mental health setting. However, the type of position would vary according to the training and experience required to complete the role. As the CCGs largely commission mental health services for their local communities, the types of services would depend on the population needs. However, it can be stipulated that most CCGs will have access to or the ability to refer to a neighbouring service provider in the following settings.

Types of mental health providers

Formal and informal providers

Care is often divided into formal, e.g. organisations, and informal, e.g. family care provision. It is recognised that most care is provided through informal care. Support for such individuals is offered by voluntary, government or independent sector organisations. While this does enable patient choice, it can often be restricted by affordability.

Statutory service provision
Statutory care services provide the majority of formal care and are delivered by the NHS and local authorities. This could include voluntary counselling organisations or NHS psychological therapy services.

Non-statutory services
This includes mental health services that are not operated by the government, such as charities. Although government funding can be applied for, it can be assumed that they will mostly be funded by charitable donations.

Categories of mental health service provision

Primary care mental health
The main provider of primary care services is through a general practitioner (GP) although primary care also includes dentists, opticians and pharmacists. Primary care mental health services could include local counselling services and libraries offering books on prescription. The GP is often the initial point of contact, although some primary care mental health services do not require a GP referral. This is usually provided in the community, such as a GP surgery. Individuals accessing these services are usually recognised as having mild to moderate mental health problems, although it is important to note that the impact these difficulties have on an individual's day-to-day functioning is often severe.

Secondary care mental health
Secondary care mental health services are commissioned by the CCG and provide specialist mental health services provided in the community or a hospital setting. Such services are made up of a **multidisciplinary team** of mental health professionals to enable a recovery focus. Individuals referred to these services are often recognised as having **severe and enduring mental health difficulties**. The referral process is usually through a GP or health and social care professional. An example of this is the **community mental health team (CMHT)**, which is explored in more detail below.

Community mental health team (CMHT)
A multidisciplinary team (MDT) constitutes a community mental health team (CMHT) and works with adults who have severe and enduring mental health difficulties. CMHTs are a statutory service commissioned by the CCG. Such mental health difficulties are likely to be long term and complex in nature, with significant impact on the individual's ability to function. These difficulties are assessed, monitored and managed in a community setting, such as their home or supported living accommodation (Iqbal et al. 2014). This could be to prevent admission to hospital or oversee an individual's discharge from hospital to the community. The emphasis of the CMHT in both assessment and treatment is that of a recovery focus, rather than solely symptom management. Models of recovery focus on supporting the person's

journey to recovery and developing their resilience. The bio-psycho-social model is often encouraged through collaboration, which focuses on the whole person (Department of Health 2010). A **Care Programme Approach (CPA)** may be used as a framework to outline the ongoing processes of assessment and treatment.

As Helen states in Case Study 4.2, working in a variety of different settings has helped her develop her ability as a mental health professional.

CASE STUDY 4.2: COUNSELLING PSYCHOLOGIST PERSPECTIVE, HELEN'S STORY (HCPC REGISTERED COUNSELLING PSYCHOLOGIST)

In order to pursue a career in counselling psychology and entry onto the doctoral course, I worked as a support worker, health care assistant, research and assistant psychologist. My most notable was a split research and clinical role, which was the beginning of my experience working with older adults. As a research psychologist, I worked on a large drug trial, carrying out the assessments, phlebotomy, psychometric testing and follow-up interviews with participants. I also engaged in a large research project on premorbid personality and interviewed carers about their relative's personality prior to the onset of **dementia**. In clinical practice, I ran memory clinics, provided therapy, and designed and facilitated groups within an older adult service. The groups were centred around coping with forgetfulness, adjusting to a diagnosis of dementia, and carer groups that offered support to family members. The combination of research and clinical work was valuable in linking theory to practice and is something that I would encourage all mental health professionals to engage in. The most important gem of advice that I give students pursuing a counselling psychology career is to be confident in your own abilities and grab every opportunity to work with a wide variety of mental health professionals.

WHAT IS A CARE PROGRAMME APPROACH (CPA)?

The Department of Health introduced the Care Programme Approach (CPA) in 1991, as a way to standardise components of the assessment and treatment of individuals with specialist mental health needs, in both hospital and community settings. Therefore, when an individual is referred and accepted for treatment in a specialist mental health service care will be standardised and include:

- an assessment of both their health and social care needs;
- a care plan that ensures their health and social care needs can be met;
- a care co-ordinator (sometimes called a key worker), who is a mental health professional assigned to the individual to work alongside them on their journey to recovery;
- regular reviews of the individual's progress in line with their care plan conducted collaboratively and on a regular basis.

(Wrycraft 2009)

It may be that the individual's symptoms deteriorate and they can no longer be treated safely in the community setting. Here the MDT assessment would outline clear recommendations and include the individual where possible. This may involve the Mental Health Act for their and/or others' safety.

Tertiary care mental health services

Tertiary care services provide further specialist mental health services, for individuals with complex mental health needs. Such services are provided at a national level and thus referrals can be made between CCGs, where a service is not provided locally. Such specialist units could be provided by the independent or public sector and examples include transgender services, eating disorder service provision and drug and alcohol services. If a CCG cannot provide a particular service then funding can be applied for so the individual can access services out of their geographical area. An example of this includes psychiatric intensive care units (PICUs), which are explored below.

Psychiatric intensive care unit (PICU)

PICUs provide both a controlled and safe environment to care for individuals who present with an acute phase of their mental health difficulties. The individual may present with high risk of suicide, absconsion or challenging behaviour that cannot be managed in another setting. Such units provide specialist interventions and have high staff to patient ratios to enable risks to be minimised. Therefore, the interventions provided focus on managing the risks associated with the acute phase. This is usually for a short-term period to help reduce the risks until a more suitable placement can be found, with the aim of stepping down to a less intensive environment. These can be seen as national services and can therefore accept referrals from out of the CCG area. Such services may be provided by the public or independent sector.

THE PUBLIC VERSUS PRIVATE SECTOR

How do mental health services vary?

There is often a stark difference in provision of services in the public sector and the independent sector. Often public-sector money is used to fund independent-sector treatment, especially if they cannot provide the services themselves. While the financial considerations are often acknowledged as the greatest disparity, there are other components to consider.

Access to mental health services

The referral process is often similar in both the public, e.g. NHS, and private sectors, where a GP referral is often needed. However, waiting times can be considerably more in the NHS especially for more specialist services. Whereas the independent sector can often offer same-day, face-to-face assessments with treatment beginning shortly afterwards. Although many NHS services have defined waiting-time targets, these are often not met due to lack of resources. The independent sector often has ease of access due to their increased resources and can therefore provide more responsive services.

Assessment of mental health difficulties

The types of assessments provided in the independent sector are diverse and can be conducted by psychologists, psychiatrists and occupational therapists. While this can be also completed in the NHS, often staff work in different teams thus the referral process can be elongated. Whereas the independent hospitals often employ staff as one service, so in the same building assessments processes can be completed efficiently with involvement of the MDT. In the NHS there is often a minimum criteria needed to access certain services, such as the individual needs to be suspected of having a severe and enduring mental illness before being referred to a psychiatrist. In fact primary care services rarely employ a psychiatrist. By comparison there is no minimum criteria to access assessment in the independent sector.

Treatment of mental health difficulties

The independent sector is quite unique in its ability to provide services, primarily as it does not necessarily have to meet the needs of the local population, in line with the NHS. For example, private hospitals can provide inpatient and outpatient mental health services, across the life course, in one building. This enables the provision of a variety of evidence-based interventions to be offered in one place. Here there is often a full activity schedule provided both individually and in a group, from psychological therapy, such as CBT, to occupational therapy, such as gardening groups.

Funding of mental health services

There are various reasons why people choose to access private mental health services. For example, they hold private medical insurance or have the means to fund themselves. In addition, where a CCG cannot accommodate the needs of an individual within their geographical area, they may have to fund independent services. These are usually, however not exclusively, specialist services, for example, a PICU or inpatient eating disorder service.

Environment of mental health services

The setting of an independent hospital is often very different to the public sector. Often independent hospitals are in former stately homes, set in private grounds, with their own extensive gardens. Such inpatient units have often been likened to 3 or 4 star hotels, with dedicated chefs and housekeeping services. However, they still comply with the Care Quality Commission (CQC) regulations, such as providing ligature-free environments. By contrast NHS inpatient units can appear clinical and sterile environments, with staff providing services across a larger area, thus offering a less personal service.

SERVICE USER EXPERIENCES: WHAT IS IT REALLY LIKE BEING A SERVICE USER?

While the above has explored the different types of mental health services available, individual experiences can also vary between services. It is essential that this information is captured in order to develop service provision. There are similarities in the different mental health roles and this arguably forms the basis of an effective MDT. Here different opinion between the mental health professionals is welcomed, however, a joint decision has to be reached in the individual's treatment plan.

Case Study 4.3 explores the perspective of Sharon, a service user in an inpatient setting.

CASE STUDY 4.3: SHARED EXPERIENCES OF BIPOLAR DISORDER, SHARON'S STORY

Sharon was diagnosed with **bipolar disorder** in her early twenties. Now aged 45 years, she had been admitted to hospital over seven times and spent up to 6 months as an inpatient in both the NHS and private hospitals.

My experiences in the NHS and private hospitals have been very different; mostly this depended on where I was and for how long. Things seem to happen quicker in the private hospitals, although this caused me some confusion, especially when I was really unwell. It felt like things were happening too fast. I liked the staff and got to know them well as they seemed to do the same shift patterns, so I knew who to ask what question. Although they seemed more strict at times, this made me feel safe and I had confidence in the staff. When I was in the NHS there were lots of different staff so it felt like I had to keep telling my story. I do remember getting cross with staff and getting into trouble, I was bored much of the time. There weren't the activities I enjoyed doing when I lived in the community and I often felt unsafe with other patients around me. This was over 10 years ago now so I guess things have changed a lot.

REFLECTIVE EXERCISE 4.1

Question: What might be some of the disadvantages of having mental health services offered in both the public and independent sectors?

Hint: Imagine you are a service user contemplating accessing the public or private sector. What thoughts and feelings might you experience?

Different mental health professions: what is it really like being a mental health professional?

Psychiatrist

A psychiatrist has typically undertaken a medical qualification, which takes 5–6 years and then spent at least an additional 6 years training to be a psychiatrist. Such training includes learning to diagnose mental health problems, providing assessment and treatment using the bio-psycho-social model approach, including prescribing medication. Psychiatrists usually develop specialisms, such as child and adolescent, adult or older adult mental health. On qualifying psychiatrists are awarded membership of the Royal College of Psychiatry and registered with the General Medical Council (GMC).

Clinical and counselling psychologist

Clinical and counselling psychologists have usually undertaken an undergraduate degree in psychology and then completed a doctorate programme, which in total can take 6–10 years to complete. During this time they will have usually undertaken a rotation of clinical placements, enabling them to gain experience in a variety of clinical settings. They are trained to assess and treat individuals with mental health problems and will draw on a variety of different therapeutic models to do this, e.g. CBT. Psychologists are usually members of the British Psychological Society (BPS) and registered with the Health and Care Professions Council (HCPC). In Case Study 4.4, Maria highlights key aspects of her training and career as a clinical psychologist.

CASE STUDY 4.4: JOURNEY INTO CLINICAL PSYCHOLOGY, MARIA'S STORY

My journey into clinical psychology began when I returned to university as a mature student to start a psychology undergraduate degree. Alongside my degree I worked part-time as a support worker for students with disabilities and as an applied behavioural analysis therapist for children with autism spectrum disorder. These roles provided me with my first experiences of the complex professional relationships, ethical dilemmas and great reward that run throughout my clinical experiences. Following graduation, I worked as a health care assistant and from there gained my first NHS psychology role as an assistant psychologist in a **child and adolescent mental health service (CAMHS)**. I look back at these pre-qualification roles as important times of learning, reading, testing out and reflecting without the same pressures of being a qualified clinician. From clinical posts, I took a role as a research associate in a university. With a background that included both clinical and research components, I applied and was accepted on to a clinical psychology doctorate course.

Among the many clinical, academic and emotional demands of the course, for me the greatest was starting new clinical placements in different services every

6 months, learning the skills of quickly embedding myself into teams, independently learning on the job, and tolerating uncertainty, which I now realise go hand-in-hand with the profession itself. After qualifying, I worked in the NHS as a clinical psychologist in brain injury rehabilitation and primary care adult mental health. Perhaps what I was least prepared for on qualification was the level of responsibility that I would hold as a clinical psychologist, both in relation to client work and to my role within teams. It is not uncommon to be the lone psychologist in a team and, even when newly qualified, to hold supervision and management responsibility for other highly experienced colleagues. This presents a particular demand when you yourself are still in many ways a novice. What I have held on to throughout my career is my deep compassion and care for the individuals I work with. I am constantly inspired by their resilience and kindness often in the face of much adversity. They have no doubt taught me as much as I have taught them. At times of stress and difficulty in the job it is always this that keeps me grounded.

Cognitive behaviour therapist

Cognitive behaviour therapists are trained in both the theory and practice elements of cognitive behaviour therapy (CBT). Usually they have a first degree in a relevant health care discipline, such as psychology, then after gaining experience in a mental health setting undertake a postgraduate qualification in CBT. Some CBT therapists hold an additional qualification such as mental health nursing. This training can take 5–8 years to complete. CBT therapists are usually accredited by the British Association for Behavioural and Cognitive Psychotherapies (BABCP). Although this is not mandatory, many employers expect CBT therapists to be accredited or working towards accreditation.

Registered mental health nurse

Mental health nurses provide support to individuals, often throughout their journey through mental health services. This can be with any mental health diagnosis, applying any aspect of the bio-psycho-social model and across the life course. Training is usually completed over a 3-year undergraduate course in mental health nursing, although there is also a 2-year postgraduate course available for those with relevant undergraduate degrees and experience. Mental health nurses are registered with the Nursing and Midwifery Council (NMC).

Counsellor and psychotherapist

Psychotherapists are trained to deliver a specific model or models of therapy to individuals, couples or families. Training can be delivered in a variety of educational settings and can take 4–10 years in duration. There are different regulatory bodies, such as the British Association for Counselling and Psychotherapy (BACP) and the UK Council for Psychotherapy (UKCP). Although this is not mandatory many employers expect psychotherapists to be accredited or working towards accreditation. As Becka highlights in Case Study 4.5, there are many different routes into counselling.

CASE STUDY 4.5: HOW I GOT INTO COUNSELLING, BECKA'S STORY

When I left teaching and was starting to think about my employment options, I realised that although I considered teaching to hold a lot of transferable skills, in order to match these skills to a salary I could live on, some retraining was inevitable.

Once this became my mindset, I found that there were a lot more options available to me, and also I was able to accurately assess those transferable skills and explore the aspects of teaching I wanted to transfer. Fairly quickly, I realised that it was the pastoral side of the job that I had truly loved. This may have been working with students in preparation for concerts, shows and music exams, but also was an emerging enjoyment of being a form tutor. When I drilled down further into my role, I realised it was the relationship that I really valued and cherished above all else. A chance conversation with a school counsellor convinced me to start my counsellor training.

Despite my background in teaching, I didn't set out to work with young people. My tutor for the children and young people module was nothing short of inspirational. His passion and care for the young people he worked with resonated with my own love of teaching and working with that age group, so after a few false starts in looking for a placement, I turned my attention to schools and was soon offered a placement.

Once qualified, finding any work was hard. This is one thing I wish I'd listened to more closely earlier on in my training. I found myself in that impossible cycle of being qualified and eligible to apply for counselling jobs yet not having enough experience to be successful in the jobs I was applying for. However, counselling is quite a small world and through word of mouth I was offered a voluntary position at a high school. After a year, I was offered paid employment there and now manage a successful counselling service as well as my own private client work. Would I do it again? Absolutely! With the added value of hindsight!

In Case Study 4.6, Shelley also highlights her journey to becoming a **counsellor** and how it is a rewarding career path to take.

CASE STUDY 4.6: JOURNEY TO BECOMING A COUNSELLOR, SHELLEY'S STORY

I was in my late twenties and had been working in finance for a number of years. I wanted a career change and felt that I would prefer working closely with people rather than chasing targets. I completed a 6-week 'taster' course in counselling and particularly enjoyed working alongside others from different walks of life and of all ages. I then gained a Certificate in Counselling qualification before progressing to the next level, a Diploma in Professional Studies. My studies were completed over three consecutive years. To meet the course fees and manage my time I reduced my working days while studying. I was expecting my first child during my final year and then took several years off to enjoy being a mum while continuing research and professional development by attending workshops and seminars. My step back into the world of counselling and psychotherapy occurred when I was signposted to a vacancy with a local counselling charity, which proved to be an excellent stepping stone into my current role with a leading private hospital where I work in both groups and also in one-to-one settings, primarily with inpatients. I thoroughly enjoy what I do.

Mental health social worker

Mental health social workers work with any individual, their family and carers to empower them to lead independent lives. This can be across a variety of settings and involve work with individuals across their life course. Training is usually undertaken as a 3-year undergraduate degree, however postgraduate courses are also available. To become a specialist in mental health there is a requirement to take specific modules and placements. Mental health social workers are registered with the Health and Care Professions Council (HCPC).

Occupational therapist

An occupational therapist (OT) assesses and treats individuals across diverse settings to enable them to lead independent and fulfilling lives. Occupational therapists are dedicated to person-centred practice and work with individuals on improving their functional ability, helping people of all ages improve their quality of life. Training is usually undertaken as a 3-year undergraduate degree, however, postgraduate master's courses are also available. To become a specialist in mental health there is an expectation to have undertaken a number of post-qualifying years working in mental health services. OTs are registered with the Health and Care Professions Council (HCPC).

Complementary and alternative medicine (CAM)

Outside of the NHS in the UK, patients might at some point consult one of many types of complementary and alternative medicine (CAM) practitioners in the private sector. When therapies are used instead of conventional medicine, this is known as alternative medicine (Food and Drug Administration 2006). CAM is generally considered to be the use of complementary therapies and conventional medicine at the same time. There is not a globally agreed definition of CAM (NHS 2016) and there are many very varied therapies and modalities, however there are common elements such as being patient centred and focusing on 'self-healing'. Some people also use the term integrative medicine; this takes account of the whole person (body, mind and spirit) as well as lifestyle (Fortney et al. 2010). Patients with mental health problems being medically treated might also be using hands-on CAM therapies such as chiropractic treatment, massage or reflexology, for example. Perhaps some may try supporting problems with herbal medicine or nutrition and lifestyle approaches.

There has long been a move towards integrative models of care in health care, which embrace the whole person and in some states in the United States there are now integrative clinics and hospitals that utilise CAM therapies as supportive strategies to conventional medical care. In the United States, functional medicine emerged in the 1980s and 1990s as an integrative model of medicine that looks at the whole person and identifies seven core areas of potential imbalance that have led to the development of disease (Jones 2005). The core imbalances are believed to be modifiable with diet and lifestyle and so functional medicine has become aligned with lifestyle medicine that is emerging in Europe at the present time.

The authors of this book believe self-care and an ability to contribute to the decision-making about that care is important for those experiencing mental health problems. It is however important to remember that there are potential interactions between some herbal medicines and nutritional supplements and medications. Additionally, some medications can also interact with foods and juices especially grapefruit or cranberry. This highlights the need to work with appropriately accredited CAM professionals who are suitably qualified to check for potential interactions. An example of a common interaction that is relevant in mental health is that of St John's Wort, a herb that can interact with selective serotonin reuptake inhibitors (SSRIs) that are commonly prescribed in **depression**, hence St John's Wort should be avoided by anyone taking SSRIs (Henderson et al. 2002). Therefore, patients considering using supportive CAM therapies involving herbal or nutraceutical supplementation should probably avoid self-treatment with natural remedies if taking medication and seek advice from accredited professionals who can check for interactions with medications. Nutritional therapy is recognised as a CAM therapy in the UK with a structure of voluntary regulation. It has been described as an 'evidence-based bioscience' (Benbow et al. 2017). Accredited nutritional therapy practitioners in the UK, also known as nutrition practitioners, are regulated by the Complementary and Natural Healthcare Council and they are trained to check interactions between nutraceuticals such as vitamins and minerals and medication. They can also check interactions with foods and commonly used herbs in formulations. Pharmacists should also be able to help identify any potential drug and food or supplement interactions so could also be approached for advice.

With greater awareness of the importance of physical health to mental health and very limited access available to nutritional advice through dieticians within the NHS in the UK, it is hoped that a greater sense of confidence emerges in the potential role of accredited CAM therapists, such as nutritional therapists who can support successful behaviour change with regard to both nutrition and lifestyle factors.

Additional support roles include: Mental Health Act Administrator, health care assistant, mental health advocate

These roles typically work to support the individual through their journey to recovery. While these roles do not require registration with a professional body, the introduction of the Care Certificate tried to introduce key competencies required to complete the role of a health care assistant.

CASE STUDY 4.7: EATING DISORDER, TYLER'S STORY

Tyler, aged 21 years, has recently been diagnosed with an eating disorder; his body mass index is currently 16, although it has been lower.

> I still don't want to admit I have a problem, I know the people around me are trying to help, but they are paid to do it. When I was first admitted I didn't like being observed all of the time, especially when I'm in the bathroom. I still refuse to attend therapy, I just don't want it. My goal is to get my BMI to 17 then get my section removed and go home. The support staff, nursing staff and OTs are really friendly, it's a really tense environment so its good when we have some fun.

Question: What might be some of the difficulties Tyler might face on his recovery journey?

Hint: Consider some of the points he makes about the services he received.

How do mental health professions measure change?

While there are similarities in the different mental health professional roles, there can be differences in the expectation of these roles. Often employers will want to measure patient outcomes to enable them to evaluate the success of a particular treatment or there may be a funding requirement (see Case Study 4.7). The following will consider some of the outcomes that are measured.

WHAT ARE SERVICE PROVIDER OUTCOMES?

Service provider outcomes:

- Implement local strategies to reduce the mental health **stigma**, such as the provision of public information.
- Increase the recovery rates of individuals who engage with mental health services.
- Increase the number of individuals being assessed and treated for mental health problems.
- Decrease the number of serious untoward incidents in mental health settings.
- Achieve a good or outstanding rating as part of the CQC intelligent monitoring system.
- Reduce the rates of unplanned absenteeism in the workplace.
- Meet a minimum standard of service user satisfaction.

(NHS Confederation 2011)

CONCLUSION

In summary, this chapter has explored how the roles and responsibilities of mental health professionals differ according to the setting and area of specialism. In order to understand the professional roles, the settings have also been explored, which has introduced how the multidisciplinary team works. It is essential to recognise the importance of the individual's journey through mental health service provision in order to provide both safe and effective services.

REFLECTIVE EXERCISE 4.2

1. Give four examples of statutory service providers.
2. What is a CCG?
3. What does recovery mean?
4. Does a cognitive behaviour therapist have to be accredited by a professional body?

REFERENCES

Ashurst, A. (2015) Undertaking the Care Certificate: a practical guide. *Nursing and Residential Care* 17(8): 474–476.

Benbow, A., Ralph, S., Watkin, K. and Granger, C. (2017) Exploring the current working profiles of nutritional therapists to inform curriculum and professional development. *European Journal of Integrative Medicine* 15: 23–31.

Coleman, A., Segar, J., Checkland, K., McDermott, I., Harrison, S. and Peckham S. (2015) Leadership for health commissioning in the new NHS. *Journal of Health Organization and Management* 29(1): 75–91.

Department of Health (2010) *Responsibility and accountability: moving on for new ways of working, to a creative, capable workforce. Best practice guidance.* London: Department of Health.

Ekers, D. and Webster, L. (2012) An overview of the effectiveness of psychological therapy for depression and stepped-care service delivery models. *Journal of Research in Nursing* 18(2): 171–184.

Food and Drug Administration (2006) Complementary and alternative medicine products and their regulation by the Food and Drug Administration, December. US Department of Health and Human Services. www.fda.gov/downloads/RegulatoryInformation/Guidances/UCM145405.pdf (accessed 22 May 2018).

Fortney, L., Rakel, D., Rindfleisch, J. and Mallory, J. (2010) Introduction to integrative primary care: the health-oriented clinic. *Primary Care* 37(1): 1–12.

Hayden, J. (2011) Clinical commissioning groups in the new system. *British Journal of Healthcare Management* 17(11): 512–515.

Henderson, L., Yue, Q., Bergquist, C., Gerden, B. and Arlett, P. (2002) St John's Wort (Hypericum perforatum): drug interactions and clinical outcomes. *British Journal of Clinical Pharmacology* 54(4): 349–356.

Iqbal, N., Rees, M. and Backer, C. (2014) Decision making, responsibility and accountability in community mental health teams. *Mental Health Practice* 17(7): 26–28.

Jones, D. S. (ed.) (2005) *Textbook of functional medicine.* Gig Harbor, WA: Institute for Functional Medicine.

National Health Service (NHS) (2016) Complementary and alternative medicine. www.nhs.uk/Livewell/complementary-alternative-medicine/Pages/complementary-alternative-medicines.aspx (accessed 30 April 2018).

National Institute for Health and Clinical Excellence (2011) *Common mental health disorders: identification and pathways to care*. London: NICE.

NHS Confederation (2011) First year study of IAPT initiative reveals key insights. https://www.nhsconfed.org/-/media/Confederation/Files/Publications/Documents/Briefing_217_Talking_therapies.pdf (accessed 18 August 2011).

Richards, D. A. and Borglin, G. (2011) Implementation of psychological therapies for anxiety and depression in routine practice: two-year prospective cohort study. *Journal of Affective Disorders* 133(1–2): 51–60.

Richards, D. A., Bower, P., Pagel, C., Weaver, A., Utley, M., Cape, J., Pilling, S., Lovell, K., Gilbody, S., Leibowitz, J., Owens, L., Paxton, R., Hennessy, S., Simpson, A., Gallivan, S., Tomson, D. and Vasilakis, C. (2012) Delivering stepped care: an analysis of implementation in routine practice. *Implementation Science* 7(1): 3.

Von Korff, M. and Goldberg, D. (2001) Improving outcomes in depression. *British Medical Journal* 323(7319): 948–949.

Williams, C. H. J. (2015) Improving access to psychological therapies (IAPT) and treatment outcomes: epistemological assumptions and controversies. *Journal of Psychiatric Mental Health Nursing* 22: 344–351.

World Health Organization (2008) *The global burden of disease: 2004 update*. Geneva, Switzerland: World Health Organization.

Wrycraft, N. (2009) *Introduction to mental health nursing*. Maidenhead, UK: McGraw-Hill Open University Press.

5 MENTAL HEALTH DIAGNOSTIC CRITERIA

JO AUGUSTUS

─────────────── LEARNING OBJECTIVES ───────────────

After studying this chapter you will be able to:

- consider the different types of diagnostic criteria used by mental health professionals;
- understand the bio-psycho-social model and how it influences diagnosis.

INTRODUCTION

It is widely recognised that there are two psychiatric classification systems that are used in routine clinical practice. These are, first, the *International Classification of Diseases* (ICD), published by the World Health Organisation and, second, the *Diagnostic and Statistical Manual of Mental Disorders* (DSM), published by the American Psychiatric Association. These are updated regularly so it is important you refer to the most recently published version; at the time of writing, ICD-10 or version 10 and DSM-V or version 5 are both currently in operation.

This chapter will explore both the context and the relevance of DSM-V and ICD-10 to clinical practice, including the history of diagnostic criteria, the assessment process and in relation to the actual diagnosis of **anxiety** and mood disorders. The contested nature of **mental health** diagnoses will also be considered.

MENTAL HEALTH AND THE BIO-PSYCHO-SOCIAL MODEL

There exists much debate surrounding the term 'disorder' and whether it is best understood from the perspective of bio-medical, psychological or social models. Such approaches provide a valuable frame of reference for understanding a mental health condition, although it is important to acknowledge it involves some assumptions and value judgements.

The importance of considering both psychological and social components, in conjunction with bio-medical traditions, in the context of mental health has long been contested. In 1977 Engel argued that the bio-medical position was no longer sufficient, as it focused on a biochemistry or physiological explanation for the onset of physical well-being. Such a reductionist approach views both the psychological and social factors as unimportant. As a consequence, individuals may not be given an appropriate diagnosis and subsequent treatment plan.

The bio-psycho-social model recognises the biological or bio-medical, psychological and social components that impact both on the physical and **psychological well-being** of an individual (Engel 1977). The model enables both assessment and treatment from the perspective of the individual and a combination of the bio-medical, psychological and social (Engel 1980). Figure 5.1 depicts some of the components of the bio-psycho-social model from the perspective of health and illness, more specifically in reference to chronic pain (Gatchel et al. 2007).

Figure 5.1 shows the complex interactions between all the processes involved in chronic pain. Here the interaction between the biological, psychological and social can be examined. Such an approach can be used to gain an understanding of the individual's perception and response to their health. Thus, it may be easier to consider this as a conceptual guiding framework, rather than an approach that aims to understand all physical and psychological difficulties. In clinical practice, this can offer a collaborative way to work with a client's unfolding past and present, which Case Study 5.1 explores.

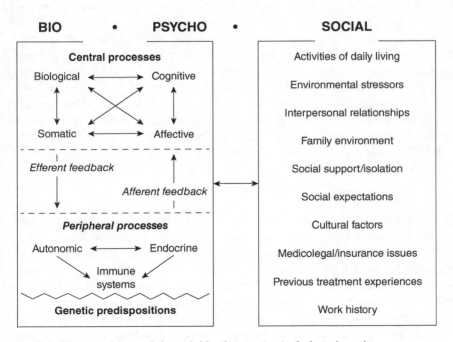

Figure 5.1 Bio-psycho-social model in the context of chronic pain.

Source: Gatchel et al. (2007), reproduced with permission of the American Psychological Association.

CASE STUDY 5.1: MEL'S STORY

In her early twenties Mel started using medication to stay awake, which she got from a friend of a friend in her second year studying at university. She began taking a low dosage, but then quickly started doubling it. Mel quickly found herself struggling to keep up with her academic work as well as maintaining her busy social life. The medication enabled her to keep awake during the night, so she could complete her university assignments and then attend a full day of lectures the next day. She also found herself feeling homesick while living in university accommodation and began studying for long hours to keep herself busy. This resulted in her seeing her friends less often as she studied for longer hours. As a child she had learnt to cope with her parents' arguments by studying for long hours and gained their praise after achieving good grades.

At university her lecturers began congratulating her on her progress and the high grades that she was achieving. Mel continued to use the stay-awake medication and work long hours throughout her studies and she achieved a first-class honours degree. She subsequently gained a graduate job in a law firm. Mel began taking a stronger stay-awake medication in order to enable her to complete her work both day and night. Mel noticed she was becoming increasingly fatigued at work and was not keeping up with her work consistently. She had become forgetful, on occasions missing important deadlines and was late for meetings. Her line manager had commented on this, suggesting she manage her time in a better way. This led to Mel using increased amounts of cocaine, a known stimulant. In the short term her work improved. However, Mel was increasingly becoming **paranoid**, developed various physical health problems and began taking time off work. On discussing this with a close friend and then her GP, Mel realised that she was addicted to cocaine.

Therefore, when working with Mel it is essential to acknowledge the biological context and associated abnormalities that exist as a direct result of drug use. This includes difficulties with short-term memory and other physical health problems, which must be further assessed through medical testing, e.g. the bio-medical model. Such an assessment must include the impact of this on her daily functioning, including her ability to work, e.g. the social model. In addition, the meaning this holds for her must also be explored as well as her coping mechanisms and if she has access to a support network, e.g. the psychological model.

Although, it is important to acknowledge the complex interplay that exists between the bio-medical, psychological and social components of the bio-psycho-social model. Research indicates that the interface between the components of the bio-psycho-social model often help us to understand an individual's symptoms. For example, an acknowledgement that drug addiction has resulted from the interplay between components of the bio-psycho-social model. Such a model provides a framework to conduct an assessment and thus a treatment plan can be put in place, in collaboration with the individual (Shapiro, Schwartz and Astin 1996). In reference to Mel, this includes how she may have learnt unhelpful coping strategies as a child, growing up in what we might understand as a hostile environment. As a young adult, such coping strategies developed into perfectionist tendencies and ultimately drug addiction to sustain such perfectionism. Understanding the function of unhelpful behaviours can be a helpful way to find alternative coping strategies. The function of Mel's behaviour could be understood as a way of her gaining control over areas of her life that she struggles to manage (Heckhausen and Schulz 1995) and therefore, a way of helping Mel would be to help her find ways to accept the things she cannot control, e.g. managing her emotions differently.

HISTORY OF MENTAL HEALTH DIAGNOSTICS

The first ICD was created in 1893 and was named the International List of Causes of Death. The World Health Organisation became involved in 1948. The first DSM was published in 1952 having evolved over a 60-year period. It was largely developed in response to the needs of military personnel involved in the Second World War. DSM-I therefore attempted to standardise diagnostic criteria for use in the military. DSM-II was published in 1968 in response to emerging research that was conducted in the post-war period. Clinicians began critiquing DSM-II, recognising the limitations in its application, such as the descriptive nature of the phrases used. Arguably this could lead to clinicians deducing very different diagnoses for the same individual, thus reducing the clinical reliability. The two later versions, DSM-III published in 1980 and DSM-IV published in 1994, presented diagnostic criteria that was more accessible and clearly outlined criteria that had to be met. DSM-IV also included cultural variations. DSM-V, published in 2013, produced subsets of disorders that enables further refinement of the diagnosis, although it is important to note that the revisions in DSM-V have been met with much controversy. In summary, the DSM has developed over time to provide clinicians with a comprehensive guide.

WHAT IS THE PURPOSE OF UPDATING DIAGNOSTIC CRITERIA SO MANY TIMES?

This chapter is exploring the purpose of diagnostic criteria; let's take a step back and consider why it has been updated so often. DSM and ICD provide current specific diagnostic criteria relevant to each disorder, for clinicians to apply in practice. This provides a standardised set of criteria, to enable a more accurate and consistent approach to be taken by all. Thus, in theory, the same person, presenting with the same symptoms, to two different psychiatrists, should reach the same diagnosis. In addition, it allows research to be conducted accurately, for example comparing the outcomes of individuals who are being treated for a particular diagnosis. It also reflects sociocultural changes that have occurred in society and the different needs this might present. Updates also include lessons learnt in clinical practice, such as unhelpful diagnostic labels. For example, in the current edition, DSM-V, the diagnosis of anorexia nervosa excludes amenorrhea, as this fails to recognise men or indeed post-menopausal women, of which there has been an increase in prevalence since publication of the DSM-IV. In addition, criteria for binge-eating disorder has reduced to one episode weekly, for 3 months. Therefore, updates in diagnostic criteria are required to ensure they are inclusive, the longevity of diagnostic criteria is appropriate and that they reflect advancements made in clinical practice.

Why have diagnostic criteria?

Traditionally, the sciences have used systems of classification as the basis for their subject. Think about the periodic table as a biochemistry example of classification. Such systems provide us with the means to understand information presented to us, such as the cause of a particular mental health problem. Case Studies 5.1 and 5.2 demonstrate two different potential triggers: John's PTSD was caused while serving in Afghanistan and Mel's perfectionism was caused by her early childhood experience. However, it is important to remember the cause is only one factor; the clinician would also need to establish additional aspects, such as current triggers and maintenance factors. Therefore, while important, classification systems are one component of a wider assessment process.

Classification systems

There are many similarities between the two approaches of the ICD and DSM, such as the identification of symptoms. However, the organisation of symptoms in each system can lead to different diagnoses. The use of the classification systems also varies geographically. ICD-10 is frequently applied in Europe and beyond, whereas DSM-V is used throughout America and Canada. Different organisations in the UK require their staff to use DSM-V and/or ICD-10 in routine practice, to assess individuals. DSM-V does not include recommendations for treatment, however by enabling a diagnosis an evidence-based treatment plan can be identified afterwards, e.g. NICE guidelines. Although it is also important to recognise that the National Institute of Health and Care Excellence (NICE) also outlines symptoms, with evidence-based interventions. These include assessment techniques and subsequent interventions that encompass three components: the bio-medical, psychological and social models. Such assessments encompass subjective observations made by the individual, and objective observations made by others, including mental health professionals. In order for diagnostic criteria to be met, a minimum number of observations must be made. For example, as mentioned earlier a diagnosis of binge-eating disorder requires one episode weekly of binge eating behaviours, for 3 months. This diagnosis is usually completed by a psychiatrist or GP, as explored in Chapter 4. Case Study 5.2 provides the example of John, who is experiencing symptoms of both anxiety and **depression**, demonstrating how diagnostic criteria can work in practice.

CASE STUDY 5.2: JOHN'S STORY

John is a veteran in his late forties who served in the military for over 20 years, having joined up when he was 18 years old. He travelled across the world, most recently undertaking three tours in Afghanistan. During each (6-month) tour he witnessed different traumatic events, including the death of one of his friends. Six months ago while on leave, his family began to notice him withdrawing from everyday life, which, at its worst, led to him not leaving the house for weeks at a time. His family sought guidance from his GP. During this time he disclosed he had been re-living the events that happened to him in Afghanistan every day. Subsequently, he had been having panic attacks during flashbacks of past events, nightmares, poor sleep, reduced appetite, as well feelings of guilt and shame about the events that happened.

In the knowledge that DSM-V and ICD-10 are routinely used in clinical practice to diagnose mental health difficulties, Table 5.1 explores this in the context of John's story in Case Study 5.2.

Table 5.1 Applying diagnostic criteria (in relation to John's story in Case Study 5.2)

DSM-V	ICD-11	John's experience
Exposure to actual or threatened death, serious injury, or sexual violence	Exposure to a stressful event or situation of exceptionally threatening or horrific nature likely to cause pervasive distress in almost anyone	Three tours in Afghanistan, where his and his friends' lives were under threat
Persistent re-experiencing	Persistent re-experiencing that involves not only remembering the traumatic event, but also experiencing it as occurring again	Re-lives death of his friend daily
Persistent avoidance	Avoidance	Avoids leaving the house for weeks at a time
Persistent numbing	Persistent hyperarousal (i.e. heightened perception of current threat)	Flashbacks of past events, as if they are happening to him now
		No numbness reported
Persistent hyperarousal	Clinically significant functional impairment	Withdrawn from everyday life and heightened sense of threat
Duration of at least 1 month		Symptoms started 6 months ago
Clinically significant distress/impairment		Significant distress caused to daily functioning

Source: Adapted from Stein et al. (2014).

Table 5.1 shows how diagnostic criteria can help the assessor reach a diagnosis. However, it is important to remember that not all mental health diagnoses can be easily classified. Later on in the chapter we will explore differences between the systems and how this in turn can present challenges to clinicians.

Classification systems

ICD-10

The ICD-10 was developed by the World Health Organisation (WHO) to provide a means for standardising diagnostics means for health management (WHO 1992). It includes diagnostic guidelines for both physical and mental health. One of its key functions is to collate and share statistical information about mortality and morbidity. In doing so this enables comparisons of statistics at an international level and research has demonstrated reliable cross-cultural application of ICD-10 in clinical practice. It is updated periodically and published online for all to access at http://apps.who.int/classifications/icd10/browse/2010/en.

DSM-V

DSM-V was developed by the American Psychiatric Association and used predominantly in America, although its use is encouraged by certain professions around the world. It provides standardised criteria in the classification of mental health difficulties. It recognises a mental disorder as involving a clinically significant disruption to an individual's cognitive, emotional or behavioural patterns. DSM-V recognises such change as causing distress and/or impairment to routine functions. The DSM is subject to regular updates and is encouraged to be seen as a working document that responds to change.

What is the difference between ICD-10 and DSM-V?

While similarities do exist between DSM-V and ICD-10, there are many differences in the classifications (see Table 5.2).

Table 5.2 A Comparison of ICD-10 and DSM-V

ICD-10	DSM-V
Compiled by an international organisation	Compiled by a national organisation
A free resource available online	A resource than requires funds to access
Covers mental and physical health	Covers mental disorders only
A global perspective	Largely an American perspective
Aimed at all clinicians	Aimed largely at psychiatrists

Comparisons were conducted between DSM-IV and ICD-10 that highlighted significant differences (Andrews et al. 1999). For example, differences in the wording of the actual diagnostic criteria led to different symptoms being identified. Andrews (1999) developed this, also noting how the inclusion and exclusion criteria in anxiety disorders are different between the classifications.

While the world's countries are encouraged to report health information in line with ICD, DSM is being increasingly used. This risks creating a gap between international health statistics and research. Thus, as a way forward there is a need to increase similarities between the two classification systems.

This chapter has so far looked at what diagnostic criteria are and introduces some of the complexities surrounding their application. The next section will explore how diagnostic criteria might be used as part of the assessment process.

The process of assessment

The clinical assessment process has developed over many years between the various professions. A clinical assessment seeks to collate evidence from different subjective and objective reporting methods. A psychological assessment is a type of clinical assessment where a clinician identifies an individual's symptoms in line with DSM or ICD, for example. It is important to note that the assessment process is ongoing and can take place over a long period of time, depending on both the individual and the setting. The initial assessment usually outlines the key difficulties being experienced with some prediction, e.g. severe anxiety or depression that has been persistent for a period of time is unlikely to improve without some form of intervention. In addition, risk is also assessed, which may lead to a higher intensity of treatment, such as an inpatient stay. Questionnaires may also be referred as outcome measures. Outcome measures can also be used to establish a baseline measure – measuring the effectiveness of a particular intervention, which will be discussed further in Chapter 6. Table 5.3 lists the typical outcome measures matched to the disorders that are normally used in clinical practice assessments.

Table 5.3 Examples of outcome measures used in assessments

Outcome measure	Disorder
Impact of Events Scale (IES)	Post-traumatic stress disorder
Social Phobia Inventory (SPIN)	Social anxiety
Generalised Anxiety Disorder (GAD-7)	Anxiety
Patient Health Questionnaire (PHQ-9)	Depression
Work and Social Adjustment Scale (WASAS)	Measurement of impaired functioning

REFLECTIVE EXERCISE 5.1

Identify: 2–3 limitations of using questionnaires to diagnose.

Hint: Consider what it might be like answering these questions from the individual's perspective.

The initial stages of assessment

An initial assessment typically involves structured or semi-structured questions in a conversation between the clinician and the individual. This typically includes the individual's account of their presenting difficulties, the health professional's observations and additional information from others known to the individual, although the style of the assessment may vary between mental health professionals. For example, a comprehensive psychiatric assessment includes the individual's full medical notes, which a therapy assessment would not necessarily include. Table 5.4 outlines the broad areas covered during the assessment, although remember the depth given to each area varies depending on the individual's need.

Table 5.4 Components of an assessment

Area of focus	Questions to elicit information
History	What are the past episodes of mental illness, irrespective of whether they were diagnosed or treated?
General physical history	Does the patient engage in risk-taking behaviours that would predispose them to a medical illness?
	Is the patient taking any non-prescribed, e.g. over-the-counter medications?
Psycho-social	What is the severity of the presenting symptoms?
	Over what time period have these symptoms developed or changed?
Social-cultural	What factors does the individual believe are triggering the current symptoms?
Risk to self and/or others	Is there a history of psychiatric hospitalisation?
	Is there a current expression of suicide ideation towards themselves or others?

Source: Kroenke and Spitzer (2002).

Assessment and diagnosis

After the initial discussion it is likely that the clinician will have a sense of the individual's symptoms in order to hypothesise which disorder the individual may be presenting with. It is essential to develop such a hypothesis for a number of reasons, including developing and implementing an evidence-based treatment plan for the individual.

Here, working as part of a **multidisciplinary team** can be particularly helpful, as one clinician can assess the client and allocate to another clinician as required. This can facilitate patient-centred care, allowing the collaborative development of an individualised treatment plan. Improving Access to Psychological Therapies (IAPT) was rolled out nationally in 2007 and adopts a centralised approach to case management where this kind of allocation happens.

The stepped-care model depicts the services available to the individual, depending on the severity of the presenting mental health difficulties.

The model operates on the following two principles:

1. That the least intrusive first intervention (LIFT), in other words the least restrictive treatment, is offered first. For example, if an individual presents to their GP expressing high risk of harm to themselves or others, offering a book to read would not be an appropriate first treatment. Rather the involvement of **secondary care** services for an urgent assessment would be better placed. Thus, offering the most appropriate treatment first. Consideration also needs to be given to the circumstances of the individual and treatment should have the least impact by having minimal disruption to their everyday life (Sobell and Sobell 2000). Arguably, by taking such an approach resources are being effectively allocated, both in terms of providing evidence-based treatment and promoting **recovery** (Bower and Gilbody 2005).

2. That it is self-correcting, in that by monitoring the individual's progress, the intensity of the treatment can be changed (Bower and Gilbody 2005). For example, should the individual's mental health deteriorate their treatment could be stepped up, meaning the level of intensity would be increased.

For the stepped-care model to work most effectively the mental health professional needs to review progress, including the use of outcome measures to monitor progress, on a session-by-session basis. Often the results of outcome measures are collated and used to develop new models of treatment. This includes the treatment of eating disorders (Wilson, Vitousek and Loeb 2000) and alcohol addiction treatment (Sobell and Sobell 2000). However, the stepped-care model is acknowledged as having limitations. For example, individuals may request an intervention, which may not be available to them from their local **service provider**.

In order to establish the most appropriate treatment plan for an individual a systematic collaborative assessment needs to be completed. Within this it is important to establish the social context of the individual, including relationships and place of work, for example. Another important aspect of a routine assessment is to establish the risk of safety the individual poses to themselves and others. This can be completed in a number of different ways, including direct questioning and questionnaires (see Figure 5.2).

Name _____ Date _____

Over the *last two weeks*, how often have you been bothered by any of the following problems?	Not at all	Several days	More than half the days	Nearly every day
1. Little interest or pleasure in doing things	0	1	2	3
2. Feeling down, depressed or hopeless	0	1	2	3
3. Trouble falling or staying asleep, or sleeping too much	0	1	2	3
4. Feeling tired or having little energy	0	1	2	3
5. Poor appetite or overeating	0	1	2	3
6. Feeling bad about yourself – or that you are a failure or have let yourself or your family down	0	1	2	3
7. Trouble concentrating on things, such as reading the newspaper or watching television	0	1	2	3
8. Moving or speaking so slowly that other people could have noticed? Or the opposite – being so fidgety or restless that you have been moving around a lot more than usual	0	1	2	3
9. Thoughts that you would be better off dead or of hurting yourself in some way	0	1	2	3

(For office coding: total score _____ = _____ + _____ + _____)

If you checked off *any* problems, how *difficult* have these problems made it for you to do your work, take care of things at home, or get along with other people?

Not difficult at all	Somewhat difficult	Very difficult	Extremely difficult
☐	☐	☐	☐

Figure 5.2 PHQ-9 Diagnostic and severity measure for depression.

Source: Kroenke, Spitzer and Williams (2001).

It is important that the style of questioning when assessing risk is done in a sensitive and collaborative manner, including being clear about a rationale. Some therapists or psychotherapists find such questions interrupt the development of the therapeutic alliance. However, in response to local policy, many organisations require all mental health professionals to complete a formal risk assessment.

Example of a series of direct questioning:

- Have you had any thoughts of wanting to hurt yourself or end your life?
- Do you have any plans to hurt yourself or end your life?
- Do you have access to the means? (If yes, what are the means?)
- How likely are you to carry out your plans?
- What would prevent you from ending your life? (Ask for examples)

The bio-psycho-social model is a helpful frame of reference to include as part of the more detailed risk assessment. This includes:

1. An initial diagnosis that may have triggered the current risk.
2. Recent history that includes any current incidence of substance misuse.
3. Establish information from others known to the individual, including family and **carers**.
4. Identify socioculturally relevant information.
5. Establish the individual's willingness to engage in treatment.
6. Develop a risk management plan, that includes decisions that may require immediate action if risk of harm is imminent.

DIAGNOSTIC CRITERIA IN DIFFERENT CLINICAL SETTINGS

It is important to recognise that diagnostic criteria are used in many different settings, including outpatient and community settings that may not be clinical. Thus the use of clinical diagnostic criteria may be implemented differently in a non-clinical setting. For example, an outpatient setting may not have a direct referral pathway to the crisis team, instead having to refer through the GP.

Having considered the assessment process and how diagnostic criteria are used in practice, the following will outline the diagnostic criteria of common mental health problems.

Common mental health problems

NICE guidance recognises common mental health problems as including:

- depression;
- generalised anxiety disorder;
- **panic disorder**;
- **obsessive-compulsive disorder**;
- post-traumatic stress disorder;
- social anxiety disorder.

It is recognised that they impact on the way we think, emotional states and patterns of behaviour. Different symptoms constitute such diagnoses, therefore, the individual needs to meet the minimum diagnostic criteria in order to be given a diagnosis. Largely, the individual needs to have been experiencing such symptoms for at least 6 months and recognise that these symptoms significantly impact on the individual's functioning.

Common mental health problems such as anxiety and depression are organised into sub-categories, as listed in DSM-V and ICD-10. For example, **bipolar disorder** is a sub-category of a mood disorder and health anxiety is an anxiety disorder. NICE guidance lists evidence-based treatment plans in a variety of settings, including primary and secondary care.

Anxiety disorders

Anxiety is a word that is often used to report a feeling of unease, worry and/or fear. It can encompass both emotions and physical sensations that are triggered when anxiety is experienced. Although an individual describes themselves as anxious, anxiety is not an actual diagnosis, rather there are a number of sub-categories, as follows:

- obsessive-compulsive disorder (OCD);
- generalised anxiety disorder (GAD);
- panic disorder (with or without agoraphobia);
- health anxiety.

Mood disorders

Mood disorders are typified by a loss of interest, pleasure and enjoyment in activities the individual usually undertakes. This can include: difficulty in concentrating; changes in appetite; poor sleep, e.g. sleeping too much or too little; a sense of worthlessness; thoughts of wanting to hurt themselves or end their life. Mood disorders have are subdivided into the following:

- major depressive episodes;
- manic episodes;
- mixed episodes;
- hypomanic episodes.

In Case Study 5.3, Daria highlights her experiences of post-natal depression.

CASE STUDY 5.3: POST-NATAL DEPRESSION, DARIA'S STORY

I have been diagnosed with both depression and post-natal depression at different points in my life. I had recovered from depression that was treated with antidepressant medication several years before the pregnancy that resulted in the birth of my son. I was anxious throughout this pregnancy because I had previously had a

(Continued)

(Continued)

traumatic stillbirth and also a miscarriage. For me the really big difference between the two experiences was that I was very frightened to ask for help when I became ill with post-natal depression. I was scared that it may impact in some way on my baby and that the authorities may say I couldn't look after my son. I didn't feel like this previously when I had depression and had no fear at all of seeking help.

So with post-natal depression, I had a really big fear of loss and losing my child. I really felt that everyone was against me and judging me for not coping better. My confidence was pretty low and I felt I couldn't trust people. This stopped me seeking help initially and also caused problems within my relationship with my son's father. Eventually I spoke to a close friend who persuaded me that post-natal depression was very common and that good support was available. So I spoke to the health visitor, who arranged for me to see a psychologist with my son. I received one-to-one support from the psychologist and attended sessions with my son; these focused on going forward rather than looking at the past trauma and I didn't take any prescribed medication as I was breastfeeding. Over time, I started to feel better and regain my confidence.

Severe and enduring mental health conditions (SMI)

Although this book is an introduction, it is important to understand what severe and enduring mental health conditions are and how this differs to common mental health conditions. Similar to common mental health problems, there are different sub-types of SMI including:

- **schizophrenia**;
- psychosis;
- personality disorders;
- eating disorders.

By definition SMI is recognised as non-organic in origin, meaning that it is not as a result of brain disease such as **dementia**. In addition, it is characterised as being long-standing when of at least 2 years in duration and if it meets the criteria as outlined in DSM-V or ICD-10.

The contested position of diagnostic criteria

While there are many functional aspects of having diagnostic criteria in place, it is important to consider other perspectives when evaluating effective care. There exists much criticism of the development, application and future of diagnostic criteria within mental health. Specific theorists often recognise its deficiency, such as a structured assessment process that prevents what Freud demotes as 'free association'. By excluding an individual's narrative, phenomenologists viewed this as a type of restrictive practice. In other words, not all aspects of an individual's story are being included. Similarly, from a sociological perspective, nomenclatures (meaning the diagnosis) can be seen a control mechanism. By contrast, neuroscience might criticise a lack of science, such as genetic evidence.

Certain forms of psychotherapy may perceive that assessment and diagnosis will interrupt the processes that occur within the therapeutic relationship and refrain from diagnosing. They may also feel diagnosis has no relevance to the treatment they provide. Although it could be argued that certain diagnoses are not effectively treated using certain therapeutic approaches. For example, in the treatment of bereavement, psychotherapy is recommended to allow the individual to process the loss. This is as opposed to **cognitive behaviour therapy (CBT)**, which largely focuses on the here and now, encouraging the development of techniques to manage unhelpful thoughts and behaviours. Arguably CBT does not allow the processing of the loss and thus is not deemed to be effective.

The role of the media in its portrayal of mental health diagnoses also contributes to popularist schools of thought. For example, a television series that emphasises the link between criminality and schizophrenia arguably forms a negative construct. Therefore, the contested nature of diagnosis within mental health can be seen from biological, psychological and social schools of thought.

CONCLUSION

The future of diagnostic criteria

This chapter has outlined the operational components of diagnostic criteria while emphasising the importance of other perspectives in the provision of effective care. In offering alternative perspectives it is evident that there are contrasting positions and thus criticisms of using diagnostic criteria. For example, a diagnostic-centred approach might forget to take a holistic or whole-person approach, however, taking a whole-person approach might miss important details and be critiqued for being reductionist. Through taking different perspectives on the diagnosis of mental health conditions, this may in turn challenge the way we see diagnosis and continue to develop patient-centred recovery.

REFERENCES

American Psychiatric Association (2013) *Diagnostic and statistical manual of mental disorders* (5th ed.). Washington, DC: Author.

Andrews, G., Slade, T. and Peters, L. (1999) Classification in psychiatry: ICD-10 versus DSM–IV. *British Journal of Psychiatry* 174: 3–5.

Bower, P. and Gilbody, S. (2005) Stepped care in psychological therapies: access, effectiveness and efficiency. Narrative literature review. *British Journal of Psychiatry* 186(1): 11–17.

Engel, G. L. (1977) The need of a new medical model: a challenge for biomedicine. *Science* 196: 129–136.

Engel, G. L. (1980) The clinical application of the biopsychosocial model. *American Journal of Psychiatry* 137: 5.

Gatchel, R., Peng, Y., Peters, M., Fuchs, P. and Turk, D. (2007) The biopsychosocial approach to chronic pain: scientific advances and future directions. *Psychological Bulletin* 133: 581–624.

Heckhausen, J. and Schulz, R. (1995) A life-span theory of control. *Psychological Review* 102(2): 284–304.

Kroenke, K. and Spitzer, R. L. (2002) The PHQ-9: a new depression diagnostic and severity measure. *Psychiatric Annals* 32(9): 509–515.

Kroenke, K., Spitzer, R. L. and Williams, J. B. W. (2001) The PHQ-9: validity of a brief depression severity measure. *Journal of General Internal Medicine* 16(606): 606–613.

Shapiro, D. H., Schwartz, C. E. and Astin, J. A. (1996) Controlling ourselves, controlling our world: psychology's role in understanding positive and negative consequences of seeking and gaining control. *American Psychologist* 51: 1213–1230.

Sobell, M. and Sobell, L. (2000) Stepped care as a heuristic approach to the treatment of alcohol problems. *Journal of Consulting and Clinical Psychology* 68: 573–579.

Stein, D. J., McLaughlin, K. A., Koenen, K. C., Atwoli, L., Friedman, M. J., Hill, E. D. and Kessler, R. C. (2014) DSM-5 and ICD-11 definitions of post-traumatic stress disorder: investigating narrow and broad approaches. *Depression and Anxiety* 31(6): 494–505.

Wilson, G., Vitousek, K. and Loeb, K. (2000) Stepped-care treatment for eating disorders. *Journal of Consulting and Clinical Psychology* 68: 564–572.

World Health Organisation (1992) *The ICD-10 classification of mental and behavioural disorders: clinical descriptions and diagnostic guidelines*. Geneva: World Health Organisation.

6 INTERVENTIONS

JO AUGUSTUS, BRIONY WILLIAMS AND JUSTINE BOLD

===== LEARNING OBJECTIVES =====

After studying this chapter you will be able to:

- understand the emergence of different waves of psychological therapies;
- consider the different types of psychological therapies that are available, including individual and group interventions;
- understand the psychological intervention in the context of the individual rather than the diagnosis on its own;
- understand the importance of taking a holistic approach when offering a specific intervention;
- understand connections between physical and mental health and the role of nutrition in prevention and recovery.

This chapter is divided into two parts: Part I looks at psychological interventions and Part II explores the links between nutrition, physical health and **mental health**.

PART I: PSYCHOLOGICAL INTERVENTIONS

INTRODUCTION

Psychological therapy is an umbrella term used to describe psychological interventions used to treat both common and **severe and enduring mental health difficulties**. The National Institute for Health and Care Excellence (NICE) guidelines provide the evidence base for the use of interventions in the treatment for specific diagnoses. The Improving Access to Psychological Therapies (IAPT) programme implemented various initiatives that focused on cognitive behaviour therapies to effectively and efficiently address common mental health problems such as **anxiety** and **depression** in the UK (Clark et al. 2009; Ghosh 2009; Kristjánsdóttir et al. 2016). IAPT employs a stepped-care model that seeks to standardise treatment according to the perceived level of need of the patient. The patient can be stepped up or stepped down to another intervention if needed (Mackinnon and Murphy 2016). The IAPT programme for children and young people was embedded in many existing services from 2011, to widen access to psychological therapies across the life course. See Chapter 4 for further information about the stepped-care model.

NICE was established in 1999 with the aim on producing guidance for professionals in the NHS and public health communities, to deliver the highest possible standard of care (Rawlins 2011). Here it was highlighted that psychological interventions and medication, as well as the involvement of the patient, their family and **carers** as part of the **multidisciplinary team (MDT)** are all of equal importance. Psychological therapies are a central feature to most NICE mental health guidance. For example, this includes the recommendation that **cognitive behavioural therapy (CBT)** and family interventions are taken in the treatment of **schizophrenia** (Rawlins 2011). It is of paramount importance that carers are included and considered in the context of their own support needs, as Marie states in Case Study 6.1.

CASE STUDY 6.1: CARER EXPERIENCE OF THEIR PARENTS' COGNITIVE DECLINE, MARIE'S STORY

Managing my feelings after the sudden onset of Mum's cognitive impairment after a stroke, and Dad's delirium after a fall, was emotionally shocking. It brought a raft of other concerns for me as carer. The financial and practical measures of sudden onset incapacity heap pressure on to a patient and their loved ones at a time when they are reeling from the emotional earthquake and terror of near-death, and people may be feeling guilty about what they perhaps could or should have done to protect their loved ones. Finding that staff were approachable and honest about what the future might hold, both short and long term, was incredibly empowering. My take-home message for people training to work with carers and patients in this sort of situation would be – people don't necessarily want it sugar coated, and an honest, open and empowering approach can make it more bearable for both patients and their carers.

Here Marie highlights an important point about talking honestly and openly with family and carers, as well as offering support should it be needed.

THE EMERGENCE OF THIRD-WAVE THERAPIES

Cognitive therapy (CT) is a well-established therapeutic approach that is often the first intervention in the treatment of anxiety and depression-related disorders. However, in recent years other forms of cognitive therapy have developed and with it the emergence of third-wave therapies (Jakobsen et al. 2012). However, in order to understand this emergence consideration needs to be given to first-wave therapies. In the development of cognitive therapy for depression Beck et al. (1979) understood that critical life events could highlight negative core beliefs that in turn may create negative automatic thoughts and could lead to depression. Thus, a treatment approach to this is to challenge the negative thoughts (Beck et al. 1979). However, over time other forms of cognitive therapy have emerged and approach thoughts and thinking in a different way (Jakobsen et al. 2012). These techniques are increasingly gaining international recognition and are referred to as third-wave cognitive therapies (Jakobsen et al. 2012).

First-wave therapies are largely seen to relate to behavioural therapeutic approaches characterised by operant and classical conditioning principles, which may include exposure-based therapies, desensitisation and behaviour modification (David and Hofmann 2013). Second-wave therapies are seen in relation to the modification of negative thoughts/beliefs specific to cognitive therapies, which includes cognitive therapy (CT) and rational emotive behavioural therapy (REBT). Third-wave therapies are represented by a move towards responding to thoughts and emotions through noticing, rather than seeking to modify (Springer 2012). They include dialectical behaviour therapy (DBT), acceptance and commitment therapy (ACT), schema therapy, mindfulness-based cognitive therapy (MBCT), and meta-cognitive therapy (MCT) (Kahl et al. 2011). There exists a growing body of evidence that third-wave therapies are more effective in the treatment of depression, e.g. prevention of relapse as well as other mental health difficulties (Coelho, Canter and Ernst 2007; Fledderus et al. 2011; Linehan et al. 2006). While first-wave therapies remain important there is a need for ongoing research into the effectiveness of third-wave therapies.

Psychological therapies can be delivered individually and in groups, although for some the mode of delivery is dependent on the intervention and the mental health difficulty. Theory-driven approaches have seen a rise in the manualised diagnosis of specific treatments that use specific components including psycho-education, cognitive restructuring, behavioural activation and situational exposure. Such treatments manuals exist for different anxiety disorders, e.g. generalised anxiety disorder, **panic disorder**, **obsessive-compulsive disorder** and post-traumatic stress disorder (Borkovec and Sharpless 2004; Clark 1996; Ehlers and Clark 2000; Salkovskis 1999). Treatment manuals also exist for unipolar depression (García-Escalera et al. 2016).

While guidelines often recommend specific interventions for specific diagnoses, there is an increasing recognition of a transdiagnostic approach. Here transdiagnostic refers to the applications of the same underlying treatment across different mental health diagnoses, without applying a protocol to the diagnosis (McEvoy, Nathan and Norton 2009). Thus, transdiagnostic cognitive behavioural therapy applies CBT to different disorders that are characterised by similar cognitive, behavioural and emotional factors (García-Escalera et al. 2016).

The following will introduce some of the different psychological therapies available both in the UK and abroad.

Cognitive behaviour therapy (CBT)

CBT is a psycho-social intervention that uses evidence-based practice guided by empirical research to improve **psychological well-being**. CBT encourages the individual to develop alternative coping strategies. While the focus of therapy is on current difficulties, the past is not ignored. This may include modifying unhelpful behaviours and cognitions, e.g. thoughts, assumptions/rules or beliefs and problem solving (Beck 2011). CBT encourages the individual to identify changes in cognitive thinking, emotions, physical sensations or behaviours and use an alternative coping strategy. CBT can be applied in a formulaic manner and indeed this is encouraged when treating specific diagnoses. Although, it is important to note that a more individualised approach is required when an individual has more than one diagnosis. CBT is recognised as being helpful to treat both common mental health problems and some severe and enduring mental health difficulties. Although for anorexia nervosa, CBT has a limited or poor evidence base in supporting **recovery** (APA 2006; NICE 2004). Some researchers attribute this to the complex presentation that requires the involvement of different modalities of therapies as well as different mental health professionals as part of the MDT.

Counselling

As a talking therapy, counselling allows individuals to discuss their difficulties in an environment that is seen as enabling and safe. The **counsellor** may foster the core conditions to enable them to be with the individual in whatever they choose to bring to the therapy. The issue or difficulty being discussed is unique to the individual and may relate to an exploration of specific thoughts or emotions or a change in their everyday life. Unlike CBT, the focus of counselling sessions may be from past experiences or being able to understand the past and its influence on the present. Counselling has many different specialisms and as such can work with a variety of mental health difficulties, however, this is assuming the counsellor has undertaken specific forms of training and supervision. Examples include couples counselling, family therapy and bereavement counselling (Feltham, Hanley and Winter 2017). Counselling does not consistently use outcome measures that may form the evidence of CBT, therefore, it is difficult to compare the two modalities. As such CBT has been viewed as being more effective, however, it is widely acknowledged that counselling is effective in its own right. For example, the loss of a loved one may be better addressed in bereavement or family counselling to enable the individual or family to process the sense of loss. Fundamentally, there is a choice of therapies given to the individual enabling a person-centred approach.

Dialectical behaviour therapy (DBT)

DBT as an evidence-based approach helps individuals develop ways to regulate their emotions, through developing an awareness of different emotional states and learning ways to cope with these. It was developed for individuals with a diagnosis of borderline personality disorder, who may use unhelpful behaviour such as deliberate self-harm or substances as coping mechanisms to tolerate distress. Such behaviours may have developed from unhealthy attachments or traumatic incidents that occurred from a young age. Thus, DBT might support the individual to notice early warning signs of changes in cognitive or emotional states and encourage other ways to cope with distress (Linehan and Dimeff 2001).

Eye-movement desensitisation reprocessing (EMDR)

EMDR is an evidence-based psychotherapy for the treatment of psychological trauma and other mental health disorders in adults, children and young people. It uses eye movement or other forms of bilateral stimulation to enable individuals to process trauma memories and associated beliefs they may have (Shapiro and Laliotis 2010). This intervention operates on the theory that an experience that the individual finds distressing is not fully processed as it overwhelms the normal mechanisms in place. As an intervention the individual recalls distressing images while the therapist uses a method of bilateral stimulation. The evidence base has stimulated much debate and as such could be described as emerging. This largely relates to the efficacy of the research conducted (Lee and Cuijpers 2013).

Acceptance commitment therapy (ACT)

ACT is an evidence-based psychological intervention that uses specific strategies to increase an individual's flexibility. Strategies relate to acceptance and mindfulness as well as commitment and behaviour change strategies. ACT was developed in 1982, creating an approach that combines cognitive and **behavioural therapy** (Hayes et al. 2012). A central principle of ACT is to be present to whatever happens in day-to-day life and move towards a valued direction, rather than challenge or modify our responses. Here there is the possibility to open up to difficulty such as unpleasant feelings and learn to accept these, rather than avoid difficulty by pushing it away, for example. By doing so the individual can work with difficulty and move in the direction of what is important to them, their valued direction, e.g. sense of closeness when socialising with friends. Here psychological flexibility to our experiences is a central theme. There are various protocols that exist for ACT, including those for specific problems, e.g. relationship difficulties (Harris 2009) and mental health, e.g. psychosis and sleep (Bach, Hayes and Gallop 2012; Espie 2002). Individuals who practise ACT are generally trained in a profession and then undertake ACT training through CPD courses, for example a CBT therapist who undertakes annual CP workshops and has monthly clinical supervision with an experienced ACT supervisor.

Mindfulness-based stress reduction (MBSR)

Mindfulness is attending to the present moment with non-judgemental awareness (Kabat-Zinn 1996). Jon Kabat-Zinn developed MBSR at the University of Massachusetts Medical Centre in 1979. It has since been adopted internationally as an evidence-based approach in the management of medical and psychological symptoms in a variety of settings. Research has shown clinically significant reductions in symptoms for individuals with chronic pain, severe depression and anxiety for up to four years as detailed in follow-up studies (Cladder-Micus et al. 2015; Hofmann et al. 2010; La Cour and Petersen 2015). Some of the key principles taught are based on the philosophy of non-striving, non-judgement, acceptance, letting go and beginners' mind (Kabat-Zinn 1996). Focusing on the present enables an awareness of a sense of self and the surrounding environment, in order to increase the individual's ability to cope.

Such a present-moment awareness can also offer an alternative to worry about the future or rumination about the past (Hayes et al. 2011). MBSR is traditionally taught in small groups over 8 weeks for up to 2.5 hours each session with 45 minutes' daily home practice and a full-day retreat. The formal practices include sitting practice, body scan and mindful movement. Informal practice is also taught and encouraged so participants can integrate mindfulness into their daily routine. The 8-week programme has been adapted so that it can be taught individually. It is expected that the facilitators have undertaken certified training courses and have extensive personal experience of mindfulness-based practice. Mindfulness-based cognitive therapy (MBCT) was developed after MBSR, combining many of the same techniques and delivered in the same way. However, MBCT integrates elements of CBT such as the identification and management of negative thought patterns (Hofmann et al. 2010).

Psychodynamic psychotherapy

Psychodynamic psychotherapy draws on the theories, practices and concepts of psychoanalysis, that include ego psychology, self-psychology, attachment theory and object-relations theory (Gabbard 2010). The therapeutic processes can act to help the individual to understand their inner experiences and influences of past or current relationships, which in turn can help resolve difficulties. There is a recognition that our mental life is largely unconscious and can include childhood experiences. Therefore, maladaptive or unhelpful coping strategies could be seen as unconscious. The individual's transference to the therapist is a principal source of understanding and the therapist's countertransference offers understanding of what the individual may evoke in others around them. Here any resistance the individual experiences is a focus, as well as symptoms and behavioural patterns that may be explored as unconscious force (Shedler 2010). This is done in the service of the therapist helping the individual to work towards becoming authentic and unique in their sense of self. Dynamic interpersonal therapy (DIT) was developed more recently as a form of brief psychodynamic psychotherapy (16 sessions) developed for the treatment of depression (Lemma, Target and Fonagy 2010). DIT aims to help the individual understand their symptoms in the context of their relationships and therefore improve their ability to cope.

Narrative therapy: re-telling and therapeutic writing

The re-voicing of trauma experience is a normal part of many therapeutic interventions for people who have experienced trauma (Kaminer 2006). This act of re-telling is sometimes referred to as 'disclosure'. While exact mechanisms are not understood it seems this 'cathartic' act of disclosure, i.e. 'getting something off your chest', can have a beneficial therapeutic effect (Pennebaker 1997). A meta-analysis of 146 randomised control studies has shown encouraging results across a broad spectrum of outcomes including psychological health, physiological functioning, reported health and general functioning (Frattoroli 2006). Other research on writing as support in conditions such as asthma and arthritis has reported reductions in physical symptoms and improvements in pain (Bovsun 1999). It is therefore no surprise that therapeutic writing is used within many psychotherapeutic approaches. For example, narrative exposure therapy (NET) is a trauma-focused intervention that has been found to be effective in the treatment of individuals who have experienced repeated trauma (Mauritz et al. 2016). Schauer, Neuner, and Elbert (2011) noted key characteristics of NET that include: chronological reconstruction; prolonged exposure to the traumatic memory; and reprocessing of the physiological, sensory, cognitive and emotional responses. These are similar processes to narrative therapy, however individuals are also encouraged to rescript the ending, which may include new information learnt (White and Epston 1990). Narrative therapy is not disorder specific thus it can be offered to individuals with different diagnoses and across the life course, which is reflected in current research (Burgin and Gibbons 2016). It is interesting that creative writing is also now being used as therapy more widely in health care and social care environments within the UK, for example there has been a move to use workshops on poetry for those living with conditions such as **dementia** within care homes (Killick 2018).

Narrative medicine has also emerged in the world of health care globally. Here, patients' stories and experience of illness have central importance and health care professionals are being trained to use the patients' stories within the diagnostic environment (Charon 2006). Patients' stories are also central to functional medicine (Jones 2005), which has emerged in the United States as a model to better deal with **chronic health conditions**. In addition, academics such as Celia Hunt and Fiona Sampson (1998) have done much to explore the role of creative writing within personal development and growth. Hence it seems safe to say that both creative and therapeutic writing have transformative potential for those using them, however we should consider that many people need professional help and support to face trauma again, and this needs to be done within a psychotherapeutic environment. Others, however, may be able to explore writing independently and health professionals should be aware that life experience can inform writing and it seems the process of crafting writing can potentially create a therapeutic effect. Transforming a life trauma using creative approaches might enable the author to reclaim troubling events and so set them to rest as a form of self-therapy. Many famous writers have spoken about creative writing's therapeutic effect. Virginia Woolf (1989) writing two years before her death in 1941, considers her own relationship with her mother in *To the Lighthouse*, saying that 'when it was written, I ceased to be obsessed by my mother. I no longer hear her voice; I do not see her' (p. 90). Woolf's mother died when Woolf was a teenager, and she acknowledges that writing helped her move on from this loss. The novelist Isabelle Allende has also written about bereavement, as she has explored the illness and death of her daughter in the memoirs *Paula* (1995) and *The Sum of Our Days* (2008). Therefore both writers provide evidence of the transformative and healing power of writing, which is also reported by other academics and researchers such as Cangialosi (2002).

It could be argued that using creative writing in this way could be viewed as a form of autoethnographic research (see Case Study 6.2). Autoethnography is regarded as 'an approach to research and writing that seeks to describe and systematically analyse personal experience in order to understand cultural experience'

(Ellis, Adams and Bochner 2011). Hence writing is a way of coming to an understanding of the meaning of individual experience against the backdrop of collective experience. Poetry in particular has long been recognised as tool for social enquiry about life history (Richardson 1992).

CASE STUDY 6.2: PRODUCING A TRAUMA NARRATIVE, JUSTINE'S STORY

In CBT therapy my counsellor wanted me to write down everything that happened to me and take it to my next session. I found this very hard, it took several attempts over the course of a week and I kept putting it off, but eventually I did it and showed it to her next time I went for a session and she read it silently within the session. After she read it she suggested I showed it to my partner as it had become apparent I had some difficulties with physical intimacy that were related to what happened to me. I did show it to my partner and he was very upset and cried. I think it really helped him to understand what I have been battling with all these years. With hindsight, nearly six months after my CBT therapy has finished, I think writing it down and showing it to the counsellor and my partner were turning points in actually starting to get better.

GROUP WORK IN MENTAL HEALTH

Groups are beneficial for a number of reasons; a primary benefit is they combat the feeling of being alone and provide an opportunity to discuss problems with others in a similar situation. There are many types of groups in many settings for people with a diverse range of mental health problems and needs. Groups can be a way to cope with the large numbers of people referred to access psychological therapy for common mental health problems. Groups are also effective in countering social exclusion for people with severe and enduring mental health problems. Thimm and Antonsen (2014) suggest that group work should be considered and evaluated in comparison with individual therapies in depression and anxiety. Unfortunately, group work approaches have a relatively poor evidence base (Carrera et al. 2016; McDermott 2003), possibly because 'groups are extraordinarily complex phenomena, characterised by constant change, action and re-action' (McDermott 2003). However, Carrera et al. (2016) found the 10% dropout rate from their groups was significantly less than the 25% dropout rate suggested for individual CBT (Hans and Hiller 2013).

Meeting and assessing group members

It is good for a group facilitator to meet group members before the group starts. This could be an informal meeting, introductory interview or formal initial assessment. The meeting allows the facilitator to consider each individual's suitability for the group.

Potential group members can also decide whether the group is right for them. It may sometimes be necessary to offer individual work rather than group work. Nilsen and colleagues (2015) reported challenges in choosing patients with first-episode psychosis who could work together well in a group setting. This initial meeting is also the start of the health professional's relationship with the individual and provides the first opportunity to build rapport. The group information needs to be communicated in an understandable way (Nilsen 2015). Group members are more likely to turn up for the first meeting if they have already met someone who will be facilitating the group (Williams 2014).

REFLECTIVE EXERCISE 6.1

What do you imagine are the fears of a person with mental health problems before coming to a group?

- Fear of being seen as different by others.
- Fears about the number of people in the group.
- Fear of being the 'worst'.
- Fear of other group members' behaviour.
- Fears linked to their previous experience of groups.
- Fear of being rejected by other group members.
- Fear of being judged.
- Fear of confessing embarrassing experiences or thoughts (Burton, Pavord and Williams 2014).

Preparing clients for a group

Many of the fears a prospective group member has can be allayed by good planning prior to a group commencing. The preparation for a group starts some time before the group commences and may include assessment, emails, letters or phone calls, booking rooms, buying resources and finally setting up the group room (Burton et al. 2014). It is an important and sometimes forgotten component. Benson (2010) points out many groups do not get off the ground due to the lack of planning and organisation. When groups are run regularly and there is a system in place for planning them, they tend to run smoothly and the benefits for group members with mental health problems are clear (Burton et al. 2014).

Facilitation and leadership

The leadership and facilitation style of the group will be based on the type of group, the leader's knowledge and training and also their values and personality. Lindsay and Orton (2011) suggest personal awareness and sensitivity are essential for good facilitation. The group facilitator is responsible for ensuring that the start of the group reassures participants that this current group experience will be positive and supportive (Burton et al. 2014).

Type of group

Groups can be long or short term, they are usually time limited but could be ongoing (Preston-Shoot 2007). Ongoing, open groups could be open to new group members; time-limited groups are usually closed groups with the same group of people starting in the first group and expected to stay for the duration. Closed groups offer more opportunity for building trust and provide an environment for sharing difficult experiences. Open groups can offer ongoing support, however group members may become dependent on the group and not seek support in other social networks. The type of activity chosen within the group needs to be appropriate for the type of group and the theoretical framework of the group (Burton et al. 2014) (see Table 6.1).

Table 6.1 The different types of groups

Type of group	Description of group	Examples of groups
Therapy groups/group psychotherapy	These groups have an overlying theoretical approach (transactional analysis, Gestalt, psychodrama) and it is important when running this type of group that the facilitators are trained and have a clear understanding of the chosen theoretical model and mental health problems	These groups may include cognitive therapy groups. Psychotherapy and psychodynamic groups can include transactional analysis groups, Gestalt groups, psychodrama groups and projective art groups
Counselling groups	Helpful for people who are finding it difficult to cope with life's challenges Useful for resolving problems and preventing the development of problems	There are various approaches that may be used. Some therapists are trained in an integrative approach or a cognitive behavioural approach
Psycho-education groups or educational groups	Psycho-education groups focus on gaining information and knowledge and tend to be more structured than other groups. They use strategies from an educational and cognitive behavioural approach	Drug and alcohol education groups with the aim of increasing people's awareness of the psychological, physical and biological effects. Anxiety-management or mood-mastery groups may also have a predominantly psycho-educational approach
Personal growth groups	Some groups in the community have aims to increase social interaction, for participants to gain social contact and interaction. The groups are often open groups with no set beginning or end session	Pottery groups, art groups, cooking groups, budgeting groups, indoor and outdoor groups

Developmental skills groups	These groups aim to work on skill development where group members work to increase life skills or academic skills	Activity groups may involve art, music, cookery, pottery or sport
Support groups	Support groups may include gaining support for an illness or a loss such as coping with the death of a loved one. These groups are most likely open groups where group members can join at any time and participate in as many sessions as they need to. It is common for people to dip in and out of the group as they feel the need, rather than commit to a set number of sessions	Gaining support regarding a specific mental health condition facilitated by people with knowledge of the condition Bereavement groups Crisis intervention groups in a community setting following a crisis or disaster

Source: adapted from Burton et al. (2014).

Managing group processes

Group processes refer to how interpersonal relationships between group members develop and change over the course of therapy (Lindsay and Orton 2011). Tuckman (1965) proposed four stages of group development, which are outlined in Table 6.2.

Table 6.2 Proposed four stages of group development

Stage of group	Description
Forming	In the first stage, the forming of the group takes place. The individual's behaviour is driven by a desire to be accepted by the others, and avoids controversy or conflict
Storming	Group members open up to each other and confront each other's ideas and perspectives. In some cases, storming can be resolved quickly. In others, the group never moves past this stage
Norming	All members agree on a common goal. Some may have to give up their own ideas for the group to function
Performing	The group is able to handle the decision-making process independently. In 1977, a fifth and final stage was added called the 'adjourning' stage, which involves completing the task and breaking up the group (Tuckman and Jensen 1977)

Source: Adapted from Williams (2014).

Burton et al. (2014) have categorised these stages according to the beginning, middle and ending of the group.

Beginning

The processes of forming and storming occur at the beginning of the group. In the first session, it is normal for participants to feel anxious. The members of the group are new to each other, and unsure of the purpose of the group. Working together to create rules for the group is a good way of commencing a group and helping group participants to build trust. Rules could be written on a large piece of flipchart paper and pinned on the wall each week or typed up and then given out to group members the following week.

REFLECTIVE EXERCISE 6.2

What rules would you contribute for a group?

Here are some of the rules that group members suggest:

- Respect the need for confidentiality.
- Everybody is important.
- Try not to judge people's behaviour.
- It's important to turn up to the group.
- You can make mistakes.
- It's OK not to know the answers.
- It's OK to ask for help.
- Turn mobile phones off.

If a group leader is too directive at this stage, it may result in group members only relating to the leader and not each other and may slow down the process of the group. The leader may be challenged by group members as they become more familiar with each other. Additionally, personality clashes and differences of opinion are likely to occur. Although storming is an uncomfortable stage, it could be argued that individuals can never truly have an honest and trusting relationship unless they allow themselves to disagree (Burton et al. 2014).

Middle

During the middle stage and following the storming stage, the group begins to find a common focus, both as a result of the ideas that have been discussed during the storming stage and because the group wants to move away from this difficult stage (Burton et al. 2014).

Ending

The concluding stage may happen when members leave the group. The individual group members look back on and review past events, and look forward with excitement and fear to future challenges. At this stage, it is natural to experience negative feelings towards the group as a way of coping and feeling better about leaving. The facilitator should prepare group members for the final stage during the group (Burton et al. 2014).

Theoretical framework

A theoretical framework is a way of understanding the individual group members' problems (see Table 6.3). It is also a way of constructing the group activities and directing the facilitator responses (Burton et al. 2014).

Table 6.3 Theoretical frameworks applied to groups

Theoretical framework	Type of group	Description of group
Psychodynamic	Any type of creative group, for example an art group, pottery group, music group, creative writing group	'Childhoods and later experiences are recreated as emotional tensions in the context of the group and its leader' (Preston-Shoot 2007, p. 64)
Humanistic	Self-esteem group	'Emphasise human emotional development and the power of the group to facilitate the release of feelings and the achievement of personal growth' (Preston-Shoot 2007, p. 64)
Cognitive	Coping with feelings group Improve your mood group	Understanding the relationship between feelings and thoughts, analysing deep-seated beliefs and their impact on self-image
Cognitive behavioural group	Anxiety-management group	Understanding the interconnection of thinking and feeling on behaviours. Understanding the physical signs of anxiety, explaining fight and flight and helping group members challenge negative thinking patterns and set realistic goals
Behavioural	Social skills group Domestic skills group Budgeting skills group	Using positive reinforcement and sometimes negative reinforcement to shape behaviour. Setting behavioural goals for change. Role-play is also used to practice new behaviours in a safe group environment. Relaxation may be used to reduce physiological symptoms of anxiety
Transactional analysis	Coping with feelings group Healthy relationships group	Explaining transactional analysis theory to group members and using the theory to help analyse group members' patterns of transactions with themselves (intrapersonal communication) and others (interpersonal communication)

Source: Adapted from Burton et al. (2014).

REFLECTIVE EXERCISE 6.3 COPING WITH CHALLENGES IN GROUPS

Think of a time when you have been aware of a problem within a group.

What were the components of the problem?

When you are experiencing problems in groups ask yourself:

- When is it a problem? Could it be uncomfortable, but productive?
- To whom is it a problem? Is it only the facilitator or to others?
- Why is the problem occurring? Is it caused by the activity, the environment, the leader's approach? Is the cause held within the group?

Problems in groups could just be situations that we have not expected or planned for so they make us uncomfortable (Lindsay and Orton 2011). However, it is important to deal with the events effectively as they could become bigger problems and make individuals' behaviours more entrenched and defensive. Nilsen et al. (2015) found the challenges could be classified into six categories: motivating patients to participate, selecting participants, choosing group format, preserving patient independence, adherence to protocol and fostering good problem solving.

Some of the problems that can occur in groups are in relation to:

The environment
In the planning stage one of the early considerations is finding a suitable room to run the group. The size of the room, access to the room, lighting, temperature and the level of noise around the room are important factors. The room size, layout and furniture need to accommodate the type of group; for example the room would be set out in a different way if it was an activity art group or a sharing supportive group (Burton et al. 2014).

Leadership
Leadership is an important factor to consider when problems emerge. Some of the problems are a result of poor planning by the leader. There may be a poor fit between the aims and goals of the group and the style of the group leader. The group leader may have personal problems that interfere with their facilitation skills during a group. It is beneficial to have a co-leader and a robust reflection time following the group (Burton et al. 2014).

Strategies for dealing with problems for individual group members

Silent group members
Lack of confidence or anxiety are the main reason group members are silent. The group leader needs to make sure that they continue to engage in eye contact and not ignore the silent person. It is important to note that even though they are not contributing to the group they may be still engaging with the process. The group facilitator can engage the whole group in simple activities that encourage quiet

members to participate in a non-threatening activity. Pair exercises are good because talking to one person and finding that you have something in common with them can break the ice and increase confidence. However, it is possible that the group is not of any interest to them and the lack of engagement is due to boredom (Burton et al. 2014).

Strategies
- Individual work may be more appropriate.
- Accept the behaviour.
- Talk to the person on an individual basis.
- Encourage the person to communicate non-verbally.
- Direct the discussion within the group.
- Use pairs or smaller group work.
- Consider your own behaviour, particularly eye contact.

Dominating member
Just as anxiety is often the reason for silence in a group, it can also be the reason for someone dominating the group; dominating the group is a way of controlling the direction of the group away from issues that are difficult to handle. Douglas (2000) notes that the person who sits opposite the group leader is often a potential challenge for the position of group leadership, which he suggests may be because of the increased amount of eye contact the person would get in that position in the circle. Scrutiny from the leader gaze may make the person louder and more aggressive (Burton et al. 2014).

Strategies
- Talk to the person on an individual basis.
- The group leader should sit next to the person, thereby reducing eye contact and allowing light physical contact to discourage them from offering opinion again.
- Direct and draw other members into the discussion.
- Encourage the person to help other members to say more.
- Encourage group members to take responsibility.

Angry/distressed group member
Anger is a way of coping when feeling exposed or threatened. Anger is a familiar bad feeling to some and feels safer than the feeling that is more appropriate for the situation. The biological explanation suggests that we are angry when we or a significant other are threatened or in order to meet our basic needs or to protect our space (Burton et al. 2014).

Strategies
- Listen.
- Manage your own feelings.
- Consider the specific needs of the person concerned.
- Encourage constructive expression of emotion.
- Talk to the person on an individual basis.
- Attend to other group members.

Disruptive behaviour

There are many reasons for disruptive behaviour. One of the primary considerations for the group facilitators should be if the person is mentally well enough to attend the group. You may see people with bizarre or unpredictable behaviour due to their mental health condition. The group member or members might feel coerced into the group and don't want to be there. They might feel uncomfortable with the subject matter or angry with a decision that is being made on their behalf. They might be testing the leader out to see how they will react or be challenging other members of the group for the role of 'top dog' (Burton et al. 2014).

Strategies
- Set clear expectations at the beginning of the group.
- Manage the behaviour.
- Speak to the group member one to one.
- Attend to the degree of stimulation (quiet environment, simple activity).
- Attendance at some groups may not be appropriate.

Strategies to deal with difficult situations affecting whole groups

Group work involves a high degree of unpredictability and this may be the factor that attracts you or puts you off facilitating groups. Over-controlling groups often leads to problems that affect the whole group. A group leader's ability to be flexible is important. They need to have a number of activities and plans in case the one that has been chosen is not going to work. The most obvious reason for problems affecting whole group is that the group aim is not a good match for the individual group members' needs (Burton et al. 2014).

A group in conflict

This occurs naturally in groups and is often the storming stage. Be aware of benefits of a 'storming' experience; it is important to discuss and be honest about the 'elephant in the room'. Group members need to be supported to experience healthy expression of feelings in a safe environment (Burton et al. 2014).

Silent group

If the group is silent it may be because they feel unsafe; if this is the case it is important to reflect on your leadership style and your preparation for the group. If group leaders appear unprepared it is natural to doubt their ability to look after you.

Strategies
- Wait – see if the group responds. If you are a new leader your own anxiety may push you to intervene too quickly.
- Allow the silence – this can be hard, but silence could be productive; it is thinking time.
- Examine your own response to the silence.
- Adapt the activity.

Apathetic group

If the group is apathetic they may be bored with the activity and the aims of the group may not be a good fit for their needs. The environment needs to be considered; is the room too hot? Are you running the group straight after a large meal? As said previously, flexibility in group facilitation is imperative so always have a plan B and if the group is apathetic, maybe an active fun activity is necessary (Burton et al. 2014).

Strategies
* Examine your own behaviour and leadership style.
* Change the activity.
* Use trust building and cohesive exercises.

Group reflection, evaluation and supervision

Following each group, facilitators should discuss how the session could be improved next time and any changes that may need to occur for the following session. Each group facilitator will have a slightly different view of what has occurred. They will have noticed different nonverbal behaviours and issues communicated by participants in the group. It is very useful for the development of facilitation skills and the support of the facilitators to have regular supervision from a person outside of the group.

CONCLUSION

This chapter has provided an overview of a variety of evidence-based interventions and those with emerging evidence bases used in the treatment of mental health difficulties. The common themes that have emerged include the importance of taking a holistic approach that builds on the individual's strengths as part of their recovery. Here a **person-centred care** is essential and one that requires the involvement of all those involved in the care of the individual where applicable, although this largely depends on the setting in which the individual is receiving support, e.g. community or inpatient services. The processes involved in many of the therapeutic approaches could be seen as challenging for the individual and therefore ensuring a joined-up approach is of great importance.

REFERENCES

Allende, I. (1995) *Paula*. London: Harper Collins.

Allende, I. (2008) *The sum of our days*. London: Harper Perennial.

American Psychiatric Association (2006) Practice guideline for the treatment of patients with eating disorders (3rd ed.). *American Journal of Psychiatry* 163(Suppl.): 1–54.

Bach, P., Hayes, S. C. and Gallop, R. (2012) Long-term effects of brief acceptance and commitment therapy for psychosis. *Behavior Modification* 36: 165–181.

Beck, A. T., Rush, A. J., Shaw, B. F. and Emery, G. (1979) Cognitive therapy of depression. *Australian and New Zealand Journal of Psychiatry* 36: 275–278.

Beck, J. S. (2011) *Cognitive behavior therapy: basics and beyond* (2nd ed.). New York: Guilford Press.

Benson, J. F. (2010) *Working creatively with groups* (3rd ed.). London: Routledge.

Borkovec, T. D. and Sharpless, B. (2004) Generalized anxiety disorder: bringing cognitive behavioral therapy into the valued present. In S. Hayes, V. Follette and M. Linehan (eds), *New directions in behavior therapy*. New York: Guilford Press.

Bovsun, M. (1999) Writing relieves asthma, arthritis pain. *Med Serv Med News* 13 April. www.medserv.dk/health/1999/04/14/story01.htm.

Burton, M., Pavord, E. and Williams, B. (2014) *An introduction to child and adolescent mental health*. London: Sage.

Burgin, E. and Gibbons, M. (2016) 'More life, not less': using narrative therapy with older adults with bipolar disorder. *Adultspan Journal* 15(1): 49–61.

Cangialosi, K. (2002) Healing through the written word. *Permanente Journal* 6(3): 68–70.

Carrera, M., Cabero, A., González, S., Rodríguez, N., García, C., Hernández, L. and Manjón, J. (2016) Solution-focused group therapy for common mental health problems: outcome assessment in routine clinical practice. *Psychology and Psychotherapy: Theory, Research and Practice* 89(3): 294–307.

Charon, R. (2006) *Narrative medicine: honoring the stories of illness*. Oxford: Oxford University Press.

Cladder-Micus, M., Vrijsen, J., Becker, E., Donders, R., Spijker, J. and Speckens, A. (2015) A randomized controlled trial of mindfulness-based cognitive therapy (MBCT) versus treatment-as-usual (TAU) for chronic, treatment-resistant depression: study protocol. *BMC Psychiatry* 15: 1–8.

Clark, D. M. (1996) Panic disorder: from theory to therapy. In P. M. Salkovskis (ed.), *Frontiers of cognitive therapy*. New York: Guilford Press.

Clark, D. M., Layard, R., Smithies, R., Richards, D. A., Suckling, R. and Wright, B. (2009) Improving access to psychological therapy: initial evaluation of two UK demonstration sites. *Behaviour Research and Therapy* 47: 910–920.

Coelho, H. F., Canter, P. H. and Ernst, E. (2007) Mindfulness-based cognitive therapy: evaluating current evidence and informing future research. *Journal of Consulting and Clinical Psychology* 75: 1000–1005.

David, D. and Hofmann, S. (2013) Another error of Descartes? Implications for the 'third wave' cognitive-behavioral therapy. *Journal of Cognitive and Behavioral Psychotherapies* 13(1): 115–124.

Douglas, T. (2000) *Basic Groupwork*. London: Routledge.

Ehlers, A. and Clark, D. M. (2000) A cognitive model of post-traumatic stress disorder. *Behaviour Research and Therapy* 38: 319–345.

Ellis, C., Adams, T. and Bochner, A. (2011) Autoethnography: an overview forum. *Qualitative Research* 12(1): 10.

Espie, C. A. (2002) Insomnia: conceptual issues in the development, persistence, and treatment of sleep disorders in adults. *Annual Review of Psychology* 53: 215–243.

Feltham, C., Hanley, T. and Winter, L. A. (2017) *The SAGE handbook of counselling and psychotherapy* (4th ed.). Los Angeles, CA: Sage.

Fledderus, M., Bohlmeijer, E. T., Pieterse, M. E. and Schreurs, K. M. (2011) Acceptance and commitment therapy as guided self-help for psychological distress and positive mental health: a randomized controlled trial. *Psychological Medicine* 42(3): 1–11.

Frattoroli, J. (2006) Experimental disclosure and its moderators: a meta-analysis. *Psychology Bulletin* 132(6): 823–865.

Gabbard, G. O. (2010) *Long-term psychodynamic psychotherapy: a basic text*. Washington, DC: American Psychiatric Publishing.

García-Escalera, J., Chorot, P., Valiente, R., Reales, J. and Sandín, B. (2016) Efficacy of transdiagnostic cognitive-behavioral therapy for anxiety and depression in adults, children and adolescents: a meta-analysis. *Revista De Psicopatologia Y Psicologia Clinica* 21(3): 147–175.

Ghosh, P. (2009) Improving access to psychological therapies for all adults. *Psychiatric Bulletin* 33: 186–188.

Hans, E. and Hiller, W. (2013) Effectiveness of and dropout from outpatient cognitive behavioural therapy for adult unipolar depression: a meta-analysis of nonrandomized effectiveness studies. *Journal of Consulting and Clinical Psychology* 81: 75–88.

Harris, R. (2009) *Act with love: stop struggling, reconcile differences, and strengthen your relationship with acceptance and commitment therapy*. Oakland, CA: New Harbinger Publications.

Hayes, S. C., Strosahl, K. D. and Wilson, K. G. (2012) *Acceptance and commitment therapy: the process and practice of mindful change* (2nd ed.). New York: Guilford Press.

Hayes, S. C., Villatte, M., Levin, M. and Hildebrandt, M. (2011) Open, aware, and active: contextual approaches as an emerging trend in the behavioral and cognitive therapies. *Annual Review of Clinical Psychology* 7(1): 141–168.

Hofmann, S. G., Sawyer, A. T., Witt, A. A. and Oh, D. (2010) The effect of mindfulness-based therapy on anxiety and depression: a meta-analytic review. *Journal of Consulting and Clinical Psychology* 78(2): 169–183.

Hunt, C. and Sampson, F. (1998) *The self on the page: theory and practice of creative writing in personal development*. London: Jessica Kingsley Publishers.

Jones, D. S. (ed.) (2005) *Textbook of functional medicine*. Gig Harbor, WA: Institute for Functional Medicine.

Kabat-Zinn, J. (1996) *Full catastrophe living: how to cope with stress, pain and illness using mindfulness meditation*. Newcastle upon Tyne: Piatkus.

Kahl, K. G., Winter, L., Schweiger, U. and Sipos, V. (2011) The third wave of cognitive-behavioural psychotherapies: concepts and efficacy. *Fortschritte der Neurologie-Psychiatrie* 79: 330–339.

Kaminer, D. (2006) Healing processes in trauma narratives: a review. *South African Journal of Psychology* 36(3): 481–419.

Killick, J. (2018) *Poetry in dementia care: a practical guide*. London: Jessica Kingsley Publishers.

Kristjánsdóttir, H., Salkovskis, P., Sigurdsson, B., Sigurdsson, E., Agnarsdóttir, A. and Sigurdsson, J. (2016) Transdiagnostic cognitive behavioural treatment and the impact of co-morbidity: an open trial in a cohort of primary care patients. *Nordic Journal of Psychiatry* 70(3): 215–223.

Jakobsen, J., Gluud, C., Kongerslev, M., Larsen, K., Sørensen, P., Winkel, P., Lange, T., Søgaard, U. and Simonsen, E. (2012) 'Third wave' cognitive therapy versus mentalization-based therapy for major depressive disorder: a protocol for a randomised clinical trial. *BMC Psychiatry* 12(1): 232–240.

la Cour, P. and Petersen, M. (2015) Effects of mindfulness meditation on chronic pain: a randomized controlled trial. *Pain Medicine* 16(4): 641–652.

Lee, C. W. and Cuijpers, P. (2013) A meta-analysis of the contribution of eye movements in processing emotional memories. *Journal of Behavior Therapy and Experimental Psychiatry* 44(2): 231–239.

Lemma, A., Target, M. and Fonagy, P. (2010) The development of a brief psychodynamic protocol for depression: dynamic interpersonal therapy (DIT). *Psychoanalytic Psychotherapy* 24: 329–346.

Lindsay, T. and Orton, S. (2011) *Groupwork practice in social work* (2nd ed.). Exeter: Learning Matters.

Linehan, M. M., Comtois, K. A., Murray, A. M., Brown, M. Z., Gallop, R. J., Heard, H. L., Korslund, K. E., Tutek, D. A., Reynolds, S. K. and Linderboim, N. (2006) Two-year randomized controlled trial and follow-up of dialectical behavior therapy vs therapy by experts for suicidal behaviours in borderline personality disorder. *Archive of General Psychiatry* 63: 757–766.

Linehan, M. M. and Dimeff, L. (2001) Dialectical behavior therapy in a nutshell. *The California Psychologist* 34: 10–13.

McDermott, F. (2003) Group work in the mental health field: researching outcome. *Australian Social Work* 56(4): 352–363.

McEvoy, P. M, Nathan, P. and Norton, P. J. (2009) Efficacy of transdiagnostic treatments: a review of published outcome studies and future research directions. *Journal of Cognitive Psychotherapy* 23: 27–40.

Mackinnon, J. and Murphy, H. (2016) 'I used to think that they were all abnormal. And I was the normal one': conceptualizing mental health and mental health treatment under Improving Access to Psychological Therapies (IAPT). *Journal of Mental Health* 25(5): 428–433.

Mauritz, M., Van Gaal, B., Jongedijk, R., Schoonhoven, L., Nijhuis-van der Sanden, M. and Goossens, P. (2016) Narrative exposure therapy for posttraumatic stress disorder associated with repeated interpersonal trauma in patients with severe mental illness: a mixed methods design. *European Journal of Psychotraumatology* 7: 1–9.

NICE (2004) *Eating disorders: core interventions in the treatment and management of anorexia nervosa, bulimia nervosa and related eating disorders*. London: NICE.

Nilsen, L., Norheim, I., Frich, J., Friis, S. and Røssberg, J. (2015) Challenges for group leaders working with families dealing with early psychosis: a qualitative study. *BMC Psychiatry* 15(1): 1–8.

Pennebaker, J. W. (1997) Writing about emotional experiences as a therapeutic process. *Psychological Science* 8(3): 62–166.

Preston-Shoot, M. (2007) *Effective groupwork*. Basingstoke, UK: Palgrave Macmillan.

Rawlins, M. (2011) Ten years of NICE mental health guidelines. *International Review of Psychiatry* 23(4): 311–313.

Richardson, L. (1992) The consequences of poetic representation. In C. Ellis and M. G. Flaherty (eds), *Investigating subjectivity: research on lived experience* (pp. 125–173). Newbury Park, CA: Sage.

Salkovskis, P. M. (1999) Understanding and treating obsessive compulsive disorder. *Behavior Research and Therapy* 37: S29–S52.

Schauer, M., Neuner, F. and Elbert, T. (2011) *Narrative exposure therapy: a short-term treatment for traumatic stress disorders* (2nd revised and expanded ed.). Göttingen: Hogrefe.

Shapiro, F. and Laliotis, D. (2010) EMDR and the adaptive information processing model: integrative treatment and case conceptualization. *Clinical Social Work Journal* 39(2): 191–200.

Shedler, J. (2010) The efficacy of psychodynamic psychotherapy. *The American Psychologist* 65(2): 98–109.

Springer, J. M. (2012) Acceptance and commitment therapy: part of the 'third wave' in the behavioral tradition. *Journal of Mental Health Counseling* 34(3): 205–212.

Thimm, J. C. and Antonsen, L. (2014) Effectiveness of cognitive behavioral group therapy for depression in routine practice. *BMC Psychiatry*, 14, 292. doi:10.1186/s12888-014-0292-x

Tuckman, B. W. (1965) Developmental sequence in small groups. *Psychological Bulletin* 63(6): 384–399.

Tuckman, B. W. and Jensen, M. A. C. (1977) Stages of small group development revisited. *Group Organization Management* 2(4): 419–427.

White, M. and Epston, D. (1990) *Narrative means to therapeutic ends*. New York: Norton.

Williams, B. (2014) Group therapy: a natural opportunity for support. *Practice Nursing* 25(4): 190–194.

Woolf, V. (1989) Sketches of the past. In *Moments of being* (pp. 72–173). London: Grafton Books.

PART II: THE LINKS BETWEEN NUTRITION, PHYSICAL HEALTH AND MENTAL HEALTH

INTRODUCTION

Trends in food consumption in many developed countries across the globe are for general populations to eat calorie-rich foods that are deficient in many vitamins, minerals and omega-3 fats (Lakhan and Viera 2008). It is fair to say that nutrition has long been over-looked in mental health and particularly in treatment of mental health conditions, even though there is a large amount of research in this area. A lot of the data is considered out of date, as much is from from the early twentieth century around the time that the role of vitamins in the body was investigated. An example is a paper published in 1928 on vitamin B deficiency symptoms (Hoobler 1928). A lot of other relevant work was done on neurotransmitters in the first half of the twentieth century and Otto Loewi and Henry Dale were awarded the Nobel prize in 1936 for their work, which built on the work of other neurophysiologists.

With the development of psychiatric medications in the 1950s, work in the area of nutrition and mental health seems to have been less favoured and so research data on nutrition considered to be strong and proving causation from randomised controlled trials (RCTs) with good sample sizes has not been gathered. However, in recent years there has been a greater awareness of the relationship between physical health (particularly cardio-metabolic) and mental health with more work being undertaken in the area and some researchers now writing about nutritional psychiatry (Sarris et al. 2015). The International Society for Nutritional Psychiatric Research has also been founded, which held meetings in both 2016 and 2017 (Sarris et al. 2015). There is also the increasing popularity of functional medicine, which originated in the United States, where **practitioners** look for the root causes of illnesses rather than just treating symptoms (Jones 2005). One of the fundamental reasons nutrition is important in mental health is that some amino acids (that make up proteins) can act as neurotransmitters and that others are vital for both neurotransmitter and hormone synthesis. Low levels of other nutrients such as B vitamins and minerals is also known to be linked to worsening mental health symptoms, e.g. vitamin B3, folic acid and zinc to name just a few (Coppen and Bolander-Gouaille 2005; Cornish and Mehl Madrona 2008).

PROTEINS

The monoamine hypothesis of depression suggests low levels of serotonin, norepinephrine and or dopamine in the central nervous system cause depression (Delgado 2000), which antidepressant medication works to counteract. This highlights the significance of the role of some amino acids that make up proteins. Protein is a term derived from Greek 'proteios', which means 'of prime importance' and seems especially relevant in mental health as tyrosine is needed for dopamine and catecholamine (adrenaline and noradrenaline) formation (Khaliq et al. 2015), while another called tryptophan is required for both serotonin and melatonin synthesis (Fernstrom and

Fernstrom 2007). Additionally, the amino acid phenylalanine can be converted to tyrosine so may also considered an important precursor to neurotransmitters (Bhagavan and Ha 2011). In addition, tyrosine is also needed to make the thyroid hormone (Rivlin and Asper 1966), which controls metabolism and thyroid problems can themselves be associated with mental health problems (Bunevicius and Prange 2010). Another amino acid called gamma aminobutyric acid (GABA) can act as an inhibitory neurotransmitter (Boonstra et al. 2015). Theanine, which is found in tea (Bukowski and Percival 2008), may also have calming effects.

Plants and micro-organisms can synthesise all amino acids but animals and humans can only make some, hence others must be obtained from dietary sources and these are termed essential amino acids (EAAs). Interestingly, tryptophan is an EAA and the precursor to both serotonin and melatonin, yet it is one of the least plentiful amino acids in the human diet (Young and Stoll 2003). Good food sources include oats, bananas, fish, turkey, peanuts, milk, cottage cheese and meat (Young and Stoll 2003). The sale of tryptophan supplements was banned in many countries including the United States and the UK after supplements produced in Japan were contaminated in 1989 (Richard et al. 2009); the ban was later lifted but a precursor called 5-Hydroxytryptophan (5HTP) is more widely available as a dietary supplement. It is important to note that this nutritional supplement should not be used by those on antidepressant medication as it has a potentially dangerous interaction that may induce serotonin syndrome (Patel and Marzella 2017), which highlights the importance of receiving qualified advice about nutrient supplementation.

Besides neurotransmitter and hormone synthesis, proteins have many varied functions in the body making them vital for health. They are used to make collagen, keratin, ligaments, muscles, tendons, skin and hair and are also vital for growth, the repair of wounds, in pregnancy for healthy development of the foetus, for the immune response and are also used as transporters for processes like clotting and pH regulation. Protein can also be metabolised for energy. Signs of poor protein intake can include susceptibility to infections, slow wound healing, poor growth as well as low mood or aggression (Rao et al. 2008). Proteins therefore need to be consumed as part of a balanced diet and healthy sources include eggs, beans, pulses, yoghurt, fish, poultry and lean meats. They have also been found to have therapeutic potential when used as supplements and it is hoped that future research is expected to confirm the significance of this role (see Table 6.4 below for details of some studies and reviews of intervention-based studies on amino acids).

FATS

The monoamine theory of depression has been dominant in the treatment of the condition; however depression is now recognised as having a more multifactorial aetiology, which in some cases can involve neuro-inflammation (Jeon and Kim 2018). Indeed, a new book entitled *The Inflamed Mind* (Bullmore 2018) claims to detail radical new approaches to treating and managing depression. Inflammation is also associated with other mental health problems too, such as post-traumatic stress disorder (PTSD) (Wong 2002). In PTSD tingling can be a common symptom (this is thought to be from nerve inflammation). Hence, omega-3 essential fatty acids found in oily fish such as sardines, trout, salmon and mackerel, nuts such as walnuts and

Mental health condition or behavioural aspect	Imbalance or deficiency	Intervention	Study details/conclusions
Quarrelsome	Low serotonin	Tryptophan	Double-blinded placebo controlled, 3 g tryptophan a day for 15 days, 39 participants completed the study. Intervention significantly decreased quarrelsome behaviour in all participants. Agreeable behaviours were increased and dominant behaviours decreased in the men (Aan het Rot et al. 2006)
Unipolar depression or dysthymia	Low serotonin	Tryptophan or 5-HTP	Cochrane Review, 108 trials were identified – only two trials, involving a total of 64 patients, were of sufficient quality to meet inclusion criteria for review. Clinical outcomes assessed by scales assessing depressive symptoms. Concluded that few studies are of sufficient quality to be reliable, but available evidence does suggest these substances are better than placebo at alleviating depression (Shaw, Turner and Del Mar 2001)
Stress tolerance	GABA inhibitory neurotransmitter	GABA	GABA administration was studied in 13 healthy subjects (7 men and 6 women, aged 21–35 years) given 200 ml of distilled water containing 100 mg of GABA produced by natural fermentation and another containing 200 mg L-theanine, both tested versus 200 ml of distilled water. Tests seven days apart. Electroencephalograms (EEG) were obtained after three tests on each volunteer. One hour after GABA was administered it was found to significantly increase alpha waves and decrease beta waves compared to water or L-theanine. L-theanine intake also resulted in an increase in alpha waves, but less than GABA administration and L-theanine intake showed less decrease in beta waves compared to GABA intake. Findings suggest GABA induces relaxation and reduces anxiety (Abdou et al. 2006)
Fear of heights (acrophobia)		Theanine GABA	Eight acrophobic subjects were divided into two groups (placebo and GABA – same dose as above). All subjects were crossing a suspended bridge as a stressful stimulus. Immunoglobulin A (IgA) levels in their saliva were monitored during bridge crossing. Placebo group showed marked decrease of their IgA levels, while GABA group showed significantly higher levels. Results suggest GABA is a natural relaxant – effects seen within one hour of administration (Abdou et al. 2006)

flaxseeds cannot be overlooked in mental health as they are anti-inflammatory. Omega-3 oils are polyunsaturated fats that cannot be made in the human body so have to be supplied by the diet. They are required for the brain's structure and it has been estimated that grey matter contains 50% fatty acids that are polyunsaturated, many of which are omega-3 (Rao et al. 2008).

The omega-3 fatty acid known as docosahexaenoic acid (DHA) is especially important in pregnancy as it is needed for foetal brain development. There are now some studies linking breastfeeding and infant intake of omega-3 with cognition and IQ in children (Bernard et al. 2017). As many people don't eat much fish, and particularly oily fish that is high in the omega-3 fats, it is no surprise that there are many studies linking poor omega-3 status with mental health symptoms (Rao et al. 2008). Parletta et al.'s (2017) intervention study on the Mediterranean diet with added fish oil in individuals suffering from depression demonstrated an improvement in their symptoms. Participants in the Mediterranean diet group were given 3 months' supply of fish oil capsules with a dose of two capsules per day, each containing 450 mg DHA and 100 mg eicosapentaenoic acid (EPA). It is worth noting that most commercially available omega-3 supplements generally contain more EPA than DHA unless they are sold as DHA supplements. There is some evidence, mostly from observational studies, that lowered maternal DHA after pregnancy may be one of the possible mechanisms that induces post-natal depression (PND), though a recent Cochrane Review has concluded that there is no evidence that supplementation with omega-3 can prevent PND (Miller et al. 2013) (see Table 6.5 below).

Table 6.5 Findings on omega-3 interventions for common mental health conditions

Mental health condition or behaviour	Imbalance or deficiency	Intervention	Study details/conclusions
Depression	Low omega-3 and inflammation	Omega-3 oils	Review reports dosages of omega-3 up to 5 gm a day safe and well tolerated (Bozzatello et al. 2016)
Depression	Low omega-3 and inflammation	Omega-3 oils	Systematic review by Cochrane Reviews – 241 studies were identified, of which 28 met inclusion criteria – concludes that EPA may be more efficacious than DHA in treating depression. Larger, well-designed, randomised controlled trials of sufficient duration are needed to confirm findings (Martins 2009)
Psychosis	Low omega-3 and inflammation	Omega-3 oils	60 patients took 1 g per day for 8 weeks; this reduced psychotic symptoms (Jamilian, Solhi and Jamilian 2014)

Dietary advice regarding fat intake is not as simple as it once was as there has historically been a focus on reducing saturated fat. This advice has been prevalent for around 50 years (Briggs, Petersen and Kris-Etherton 2017). Now thinking has changed and an overall balance of fat intake and inclusion of the polyunsaturated fats (particularly the omega-3 oils) is seen as important alongside a reduction in saturated fats (Kris-Etherton and Fleming 2015). A high intake of saturated fats such as those found in red meat and cheese is associated with increased LDL cholesterol, which is a risk factor for cardiovascular disease (CVD) (Briggs et al. 2017) and we must remember that CVD is a frequent co-morbidity factor with severe mental illness (SMI). However, it is now recognised that dietary advice regarding fat intake is rather simplistic. Cutting down the total amount of fat in the diet is not recommended as there are reports of low fat diets negatively affecting mood (Wells et al. 1998), as well as studies demonstrating they may be linked to other problems such as poor appetite regulation (Martin et al. 2011). In one study, it was found that 25% of energy was provided by fat and this resulted in negative impacts on mood (Wells 1998). This is less than the 35% of energy from fat that is currently recommended as a maximum in the UK dietary targets. These results might be explained because the diet reduced overall omega-3 intake, or perhaps because it lowered the status of other fat soluble vitamins (i.e. vitamins A, D, E and K). Vitamin D is discussed further below. It seems therefore that the focus of dietary advice on fats should be on overall balance within the diet and healthy eating with the inclusion of polyunsaturated fat, especially the omega-3 fats and oils.

VITAMINS AND MINERALS

It has been reported that vitamin D deficiency may play a role in depression (Berk et al. 2007), although this is controversial as studies on vitamin D as treatment have not yielded consistent results. In the UK the Department of Health now recommends supplementation with vitamin D for all age groups because vitamin D deficiency has been so prevalent within the UK (SACN 2016). The recommended dosage is 10 µg/day (400 IU) for all age 4 years or over, including pregnant and lactating women (SACN 2016). Health professionals working with patients with **mental illness** would be well advised to check whether the recommendations for supplementation are being followed and refer to GPs for prescription of supplements. Besides vitamin D and some of the B vitamins mentioned in the introduction to this section of the chapter, there are also many vitamins and minerals important for mental health and deficiency of these can be associated with mental health problems. For example low levels of vitamin B12 (cobalamin) may be associated with psychosis, **mania** and depression (Durand et al. 2003). Also a lot of research going back to the 1960s has demonstrated a deficiency of folate (found in green leafy vegetables) in patients with depression (Young 2007). Another important nutrient in mental health is the mineral zinc, which has been shown to have antidepressant properties and enhance treatment with monoamine-based antidepressant medication (Doboszewska et al. 2017).

Some people have genetic variations, called single-nucleotide polymorphisms (SNPs) affecting processes within the body such as methylation. These can change requirements for nutrients such as folate and vitamin B12 (cobalamin). Often these lead to a requirement for an increased intake or intake of active forms of nutrients (methylated forms), which if not met might create a functional deficiency of the nutrient. SNPs affecting the MTHFR gene that controls methylation are associated with high homocysteine, which is now recognised as a marker for CVD (Kumar et al. 2017) and associated with depression in post-menopausal women (Różycka et al. 2016). Other SNPs affect genes that influence levels of neurotransmitters (e.g. COMT and MAO genes) are also associated with depression in post-menopausal women (Różycka et al. 2016).

The traditional Mediterranean diet is a dietary model that includes healthy fats in the form of olive oil (monounsaturated fats), fish, nuts, seeds, legumes, plenty of fruits and vegetables and little processed food (Bach-Faig et al. 2011). It is generally viewed as providing good amounts of vitamins, minerals and phytochemicals, many of which function as antioxidants that can help protect cell structures from oxidative damage. A recent study on the Mediterranean diet has been shown to reduce symptoms of depression (Parletta et al. 2017). Furthermore, a systematic review of observational studies published in 2018 (Lassale et al. 2018) concluded that following a Mediterranean diet or avoiding a pro-inflammatory diet confers some protection against depression in observational studies.

Du et al. (2016) conducted a review examining the role of nutrients in mental health and found that vitamin C (found in fruits and vegetables), zinc and magnesium can protect against oxidative damage to lipids in cell membranes and vital cell organelles such as mitochondria in the neuronal circuits. These findings highlight the potential role of a nutrient-dense, balanced diet containing plenty of fruits and vegetables in supporting recovery from mental illness. Table 6.6 highlights magnesium and zinc and their potential role in therapy.

Table 6.6 Findings on some nutrient-based interventions for depression

Mental health condition or behaviour	Intervention	Study details/conclusions
Depression	30 mg zinc	50 overweight or obese participants were randomly assigned into two groups and received either 30 mg of zinc or a placebo daily for 12 weeks. At baseline and post-intervention, depression severity was assessed. Results suggest zinc improves mood in overweight or obese subjects (Solati et al. 2014)
Depression	125–300 mg of magnesium (as glycinate and taurinate)	Results suggest that magnesium ion neuronal deficits could be caused by stress hormones, excessive dietary calcium as well as dietary deficiencies of magnesium. Case reports show quick recovery (less than seven days) from major depression using 125–300 mg of magnesium (as glycinate and taurinate) with each meal and at bedtime. Magnesium was found to be usually effective for treatment of depression in general use (Eby and Eby 2006)

THE EFFECT OF MENTAL HEALTH CONDITIONS ON EATING HABITS AND NUTRITIONAL STATUS

Mental health conditions can severely impact a person's nutritional status, for example reducing appetite and causing people to skip meals (Rao et al. 2008) and reducing their ability to plan, shop, budget and cook food. This may result in a reliance on convenience foods and takeaways that over time can impact a person's nutritional status. Some medications (e.g. antipsychotic drugs) can impact appetite and influence cravings for carbohydrates such as sugar (Rao et al. 2008; Werneke, Taylor and Sanders 2013) and there may also be metabolic changes as a result of medication (particularly anti-psychotics) that affect metabolism and predispose to increased cardio-metabolic risk (Maayan and Correll 2010). Some mental health conditions can also affect the palate, for example individuals suffering from schizophrenia have been found to have preferences for caffeinated drinks and **hallucinations** can also affect taste. If substance misuse issues are also present then there may be added impacts on nutritional status, as money for food may be spent on alcohol or drugs. Alcohol depletes thiamine (vitamin B1) so this is often prescribed in alcoholism as B1 deficiency cause neurological defects and is even associated with dementia (Gibson et al. 2016). Stefańska et al. (2017) have investigated dietary patterns of a group of patients with recurrent affective disorders and schizophrenia. They report dietary deficiencies of polyunsaturated fatty acids (including omega-3), vitamin D and iron. They also state that consumption of high-calorie foods has a detrimental effect on the nervous system and suggest that this is because such foods are high in saturated fatty acids and sugars, which increase oxidative stress that in turn decrease synaptic plasticity. Consumption of high sugar foods can cause increases in insulin levels (essential to promote glucose storage or conversion to fat) that result in falling blood sugar levels and it is believed these fluctuations can result in mood alterations and potentially trigger aggressive behaviour. Consumption of food that causes steadier release of glucose into the blood stream and eating balanced meals containing some protein, fat and fibre may help release sugars more slowly, thereby supporting balance of mood.

Obesity and increased body weight can contribute to lower self-esteem, which, in turn, may promote depression and mood disorders via influencing stress-induced inflammatory processes that may further deregulate the neuroendocrine system. Historically there has not been a great emphasis on formally monitoring the physical health or body weight within care plans for those with mental illness (Lawrence and Kisely 2010). The 2017–2019 Commissioning for Quality and Innovation guidance has identified 'improving physical healthcare to reduce premature mortality in people with serious mental illness' as a key target across the UK health sector (NHS England 2017). The importance of physical health monitoring for those with mental health conditions, particularly severe mental illness, is now reflected in clinical guidance from NICE in the UK. NICE (CG178, CG155, QS80, QS102) recommend a systematic approach to physical health screening and monitoring for CVD risk, particularly for individuals prescribed antipsychotic medication (as some are associated with weight gain) (NHS England 2017). They also recommend lifestyle interventions focused on healthy eating advice, physical activity and smoking cessation.

Gluten and coeliac disease

Coeliac disease is an immune-mediated enteropathy that affects the small bowel and occurs in response to the ingestion of gluten in genetically susceptible individuals with HLA-DQ2 or HLA-DQ8, causing malabsorption (Rostami et al. 2017). Gluten is found in cereals such as wheat, barley, rye, spelt and kamut (Rostami et al. 2017). Links between coeliac disease and mental health conditions have been established for some time, for example in the 1950s an association between gluten and schizophrenia was described and it was also noted that patients with coeliac disease experienced mood improvements on a gluten-free diet (Casella et al. 2017). In the 1970s studies demonstrated that a higher than normal proportion of patients with coeliac disease could be classified as having mild affective disorders (Casella et al. 2017). Makikyro et al. (1998) reported a higher prevalence of coeliac disease in patients with schizophrenia than the non-psychiatric controls (3.4% vs 0.3%). There are also now reports emerging in the literature about gluten-induced psychosis (Lionetti et al. 2015). For this reason, health professionals working with those with mental illness should be aware of the signs and symptoms of coeliac disease, which can include unexplained anaemia, fatigue, bloating and abdominal pain, among others and consider referring patients to their doctors for serological testing if they have ongoing unexplained gastrointestinal symptoms.

The gut microbiome

There is increasing awareness of the relationship between gut microbiome and general health that could also extend to mental health. This is because the gut brain axis is now recognised as having a role in regulating stress responses via the vagus nerve, gut hormone signalling, inflammatory responses involving the immune system and also via tryptophan metabolism (Foster, Rinaman and Cryan 2017). Some researchers view probiotic supplements (live beneficial bacteria that can be taken as supplements) as psycho-biotics because they can have antidepressant effects by influencing the enteric nervous system and the immune system (Sarkar et al. 2016).

Healthy eating advice

It is best to try to give simple, practical, non-judgemental food-based advice that really helps people with mental health issues to change their eating and shopping habits and there needs to be recognition that change can be very challenging for those who live with mental health conditions. A knowledge of behaviour change is required and advice could include basic information about food types that make up a balanced diet. Tips for healthy eating should include eating at least five 80 g portions of fruits and vegetables a day (the current guideline from the Department of Health in the UK). Tips for budgeting, eating healthily on a budget, practical advice on cooking, tips for planning ahead including reducing food waste and long-life food cupboard items can also be important in helping people to create new dietary habits and make healthier choices. There are many healthy eating resources available in the UK via the NHS and British Nutrition Foundation websites. In the UK, mental health charities such as Mind and Rethink Mental illness may also have some useful factsheets that can be given to patients. Myshape.co.uk is a website that contains some free resources that may be useful if giving healthy eating advice to people with mental health problems; it was developed in Worcestershire on a project for young people with psychosis and other severe mental illnesses.

REFERENCES

Aan het Rot, M., Moskowitz, D. S., Pinard, G. and Young, S. N. (2006) Social behaviour and mood in everyday life: the effects of tryptophan in quarrelsome individuals. *Journal of Psychiatry and Neuroscience* 31(4): 253–262.

Abdou, A. M., Higashiguchi, S., Horie, K., Kim, M., Hatta, H. and Yokogoshi, H. (2006) Relaxation and immunity enhancement effects of γ-Aminobutyric acid (GABA) administration in humans. *Biofactors* 26(3): 201–208.

Bach-Faig, A., Berry, E. M., Lairon, D., Reguant, J., Trichopoulou, A., Dernini, S., Medina, F. X., Battineo, M., Belahsen, R., Mirander, G. and Serra-Majem, L. (2011) Mediterranean diet pyramid today: science and cultural updates. *Public Health Nutrition* 14(12A): 2274–2284.

Berk, M., Sanders, K. M., Pasco, J. A., Jacka, F. N., Williams, L. J., Hayles, A. L. and Dodd, S. (2007) Vitamin D deficiency may play a role in depression. *Medical Hypotheses* 69: 1316–1319.

Bernard, J., Armand, M., Peyre, H., Garcia, C., Forhan, A., De Agostini, M., Charles, M. A. and Heude, B. (2017) Breastfeeding, polyunsaturated fatty acid levels in colostrum and child intelligence quotient at age 5–6 years. *Journal of Pediatrics* 183: 43–50.e3.

Bhagavan, N. and Ha, C. (2011) *Essentials of medical biochemistry.* London: Elsevier.

Boonstra, E., de Kleijn, R., Colzato, L. S., Alkemade, A., Forstmann, B. U. and Nieuwenhuis, S. (2015) Neurotransmitters as food supplements: the effects of GABA on brain and behavior. *Frontiers in Psychology* 6: 1520.

Bozzatello, P., Brignolo, E., De Grandi, E. and Bellino, S. (2016) Supplementation with omega-3 fatty acids in psychiatric disorders: a review of literature data. *Journal of Clinical Medicine* 5(8): 67.

Briggs, M. A., Petersen, K. S. and Kris-Etherton, P. M. (2017) Saturated fatty acids and cardiovascular disease: replacements for saturated fat to reduce cardiovascular risk. *Healthcare* 5: 29.

Bukowski, J. and Percival, S. (2008) L-theanine intervention enhances human gammadelta T lymphocyte function. *Nutrition Review* 66(2): 96–102.

Bullmore, E. (2018). *The inflamed mind.* London: Short Books.

Bunevicius, R. and Prange, A. (2010) Thyroid disease and mental disorders: cause and effect or only comorbidity? *Current Opinions in Psychiatry* 23(4): 363–368.

Casella, G., Pozzi, R., Cigognetti, M., Bachetti, F., Torti, G., Cadei, M., Villanacci, V., Baldini, V. and Bassotti, G. (2017) Mood disorders and non-celiac gluten sensitivity. *Minerva Gastroenterol Dietol* 63(1): 32–37.

Coppen, A. and Bolander-Gouaille, C. (2005) Treatment of depression: time to consider folic acid and vitamin B12. *Journal of Psychopharmacology* 19(1): 59–65.

Cornish, S. and Mehl-Madrona, L. (2008) The role of vitamins and minerals in psychiatry. *Integrative Medicine Insights* 3: 33–42.

Delgado, P. (2000) Depression: the case for a monoamine deficiency. *Journal of Clinical Psychiatry* 61(Suppl. 6): 7–11.

Doboszewska, U., Wlaź, P., Nowak, G., Radziwoń-Zaleska, M., Cui, R. and Młyniec, K. (2017) Zinc in the monoaminergic theory of depression: its relationship to neural plasticity. *Neural Plasticity* 3682752. doi: 10.1155/2017/3682752

Du, J., Zhu, M., Bao, H., Li, B., Dong, Y., Xiao, C., Zhang, G. Y., Henter, I., Rudorfer, M. and Vitiello, B. (2016) The role of nutrients in protecting mitochondrial function and neurotransmitter signaling: implications for the treatment of depression, PTSD, and suicidal behaviors. *Critical Reviews in Food Science and Nutrition* 56(15): 2560–2578.

Durand, C., Mary, S., Brazo, P. and Dollfus, S. (2003) Psychiatric manifestations of vitamin B12 deficiency: a case report. *Encephale* 29(6): 560–565.

Eby, G. A. and Eby, K. L. (2006) Rapid recovery from major depression using magnesium treatment. *Med Hypotheses* 67(2): 362–370.

Fernstrom, J. and Fernstrom, M. (2007) Tyrosine, phenylalanine, and catecholamine synthesis and function in the brain. *Journal of Nutrition* 137(6 Suppl. 1): 1539S–1547S

Foster, J., Rinaman, L. and Cryan, J. (2017) Stress and the gut-brain axis: regulation by the microbiome. *Neurobiology of Stress* 7: 124e136.

Gibson, G. E., Hirsch, J. A., Fonzetti, P., Jordon, B. D., Cirio, R. T. and Elder, J. (2016) Vitamin B1 (thiamine) and dementia. *Annals of the New York Academy of Sciences* 1367(1): 21–30.

Hoobler, B. (1928) Symptomatology of vitamin B deficiency in infants. *JAMA* 91(5): 307–310.

Jamilian, H., Solhi, H. and Jamilian, M. (2014) Randomized, placebo-controlled clinical trial of omega-3 as supplemental treatment in schizophrenia. *Global Journal of Health Science* 18: 103–108.

Jeon, S. and Kim, Y. (2018) The role of neuroinflammation and neurovascular dysfunction in major depressive disorder. *Journal of Inflammation Research* 11: 179–192.

Jones, D. S. (ed.) (2005) *Textbook of functional medicine.* Gig Harbor, WA: Institute for Functional Medicine.

Khaliq, W., Andreis, D., Kleyman, A., Gräler, M. and Singer, M. (2015) Reductions in tyrosine levels are associated with thyroid hormone and catecholamine disturbances in sepsis. *Intensive Care Medicine Experimental* 3(Suppl. 1): A686.

Kris-Etherton, P. M. and Fleming, J. A. (2015) Emerging nutrition science on fatty acids and cardiovascular disease: nutritionists' perspectives. *Advances in Nutrition* 6(3): 326S–337S.

Kumar, A., Palfrey, H. A., Pathak, R., Kadowitz, P. J., Gettys, T. W. and Murthy, S. N. (2017) The metabolism and significance of homocysteine in nutrition and health. *Nutrition and Metabolism* 14: 78.

Lakhan, S. E. and Vieira, K. F. (2008) Nutritional therapies for mental disorders. *Nutrition Journal* 7: 2.

Lassale, C., Batty, D. G., Baghdadli, A., Jacka, F., Sánchez-Villegas, A., Kivimäki, M. and Akbaraly, T. (2018) Healthy dietary indices and risk of depressive outcomes: a systematic review and meta-analysis of observational studies. *Molecular Psychiatry* 1476–5578.

Lawrence, D. and Kisely, S. (2010) Inequalities in healthcare provision for people with severe mental illness. *Journal of Psychopharmacology* 24(Suppl. 4): 61–68.

Lionetti, E., Leonardi, S., Franzonello, C., Mancardi, M., Ruggieri, M. and Catassi, C. (2015) Gluten psychosis: confirmation of a new clinical entity. *Nutrients* 7(7): 5532–5539.

Maayan, L. and Correll, C. U. (2010) Management of antipsychotic-related weight gain. *Expert Review of Neurotherapeutics* 10(7): 1175–1200.

Makikyro, T., Karvonen, J. T., Hakko, H., Nieminen, P., Joukamaa, M., Isohanni, M., Jones, P. and Jarvelin, M. R. (1998) Comorbidity of hospital-treated psychiatric and physical disorders with special reference to schizophrenia: a 28-year follow-up of the 1966 northern Finland general population birth cohort. *Public Health* 112(4): 221–228.

Martin, C. K., Rosenbaum, D., Han, H., Geiselman, P., Wyatt, H., Hill, J. O., Brill, C., Bailer, B., Miller, B. V., III, Stein, R., Klein, S. and Foster, G. D. (2011) Change in food cravings, food preferences, and appetite during a low-carbohydrate and low-fat diet. *Obesity* 19(10): 1963–1970.

Martins, J. (2009) EPA but not DHA appears to be responsible for the efficacy of omega-3 long chain polyunsaturated fatty acid supplementation in depression: evidence from a meta-analysis of randomized controlled trials. *Journal of American College of Nutrition* 28(5): 525–542.

Miller, B., Murray, L., Beckmann, M. M., Kent, T. and Macfarlane B. (2013) Dietary supplements for preventing postnatal depression. *Cochrane Database Systemic Review* 24(10): CD009104.

NHS England (2017) Commissioning for quality and innovation (CQUIN) guidance for 2017/19. www.england.nhs.uk/nhs-standard-contract/cquin/cquin-17-19.

Parletta, N., Zarnowiecki, D., Cho, J., Wilson, A., Bogomolova, B., Villani, A., Itsiopoulos, C., Niyonsenga, T., Blunden, S., Meyer, B., Segal, L., Baune, B. and

O'Dea, K. (2017) A Mediterranean-style dietary intervention supplemented with fish oil improves diet quality and mental health in people with depression: a randomized controlled trial (HELFIMED). *Nutritional Neuroscience* 7: 1–14.

Patel, Y. A. and Marzella, N. (2017) Dietary supplement-drug interaction-induced serotonin syndrome progressing to acute compartment syndrome. *American Journal of Case Reports* 18: 926–930.

Rao, T. S. S., Asha, M. R., Ramesh, B. N. and Rao, K. S. J. (2008) Understanding nutrition, depression and mental illnesses. *Indian Journal of Psychiatry* 50(2): 77–82.

Richard, D. M., Dawes, M. A., Mathias, C. W., Acheson, A., Hill-Kapturczak, N. and Dougherty, D. M. (2009) L-Tryptophan: basic metabolic functions, behavioral research and therapeutic indications. *International Journal of Tryptophan Research* 2: 45–60.

Rivlin, R. and Asper, S. D. (1966) Tyrosine and the thyroid hormones. *American Journal of Medicine* 40(6): 823–827.

Rostami, K., Bold, J., Parr, A. and Johnson, M. W. (2017) Gluten-free diet indications, safety, quality, labels, and challenges. *Nutrients* 9(8): 846.

Różycka, A., Słopień, R., Słopień, A., Dorszewska, J., Seremak-Mrozikiewicz, A., Lianeri, M., Maciukiewicz, M., Warenik-Szymankiewicz, A., Grzelak, T., Kurzawińska, G., Drews, K., Klejewski, A. and Jagodziński, P. P. (2016) The MAOA, COMT, MTHFR and ESR1 gene polymorphisms are associated with the risk of depression in menopausal women. *Maturitas* 84: 42–54.

Sarkar, A., Lehto, S. M., Harty, S., Dinan, T. G., Cryan, J. F. and Burnet, P. W. J. (2016) Psychobiotics and the manipulation of bacteria–gut–brain signals. *Trends in Neurosciences* 39(11): 763–781.

Sarris, J., Logan, A. C., Akbaraly, T. N., Amminger, G. P., Balanzá-Martínez, V., Freeman, M. P., Hibbeln, J., Matsuoka, Y., Mischoulon, D., Mizoue, T., Nanri, A., Nishi, D., Ramsey, D., Rucklidge, J. J., Sanchez-Villegas, A., Scholey, A., Juan-Pin, S. and Jacka, F. N. (2015) Nutritional medicine as mainstream in psychiatry. *Lancet Psychiatry* 2(3): 271–274.

The Scientific Advisory Committee on Nutrition (SACN) (2016) Recommendations on vitamin D: SACN vitamin D and health report. www.gov.uk/government/publications/sacn-vitamin-d-and-health-report (accessed 30 May 2018).

Shaw, K., Turner, J. and Del Mar, C. (2001) Tryptophan and 5-hydroxytryptophan for depression. *Cochrane Database Systems Review* 3: CD003198.

Solati, Z., Jazayeri, S., Tehrani-Doost, M., Mahmoodianfard, S. and Reza Gohari, M. (2014) Zinc monotherapy increases serum brain-derived neurotrophic factor (BDNF) levels and decreases depressive symptoms in overweight or obese subjects: a double-blind, randomized, placebo-controlled trial. *Nutritional Neuroscience* 18(4): 162–168.

Stefańska, E., Lech, M., Wendołowicz, A., Konarzewska, B., Waszkiewicz, N. and Ostrowska, L. (2017) Eating habits and nutritional status of patients with affective disorders and schizophrenia. *Psychiatria Polska* 51(6): 1107–1120.

Wells, A., Read, N., Laugharne, J. and Ahluwalia, N. (1998) Alterations in mood after changing to a low-fat diet. *British Journal of Nutrition* 79(1): 23–30.

Werneke, U., Taylor, D. and Sanders, T. A. B. (2013) Behavioral interventions for antipsychotic induced appetite changes. *Current Psychiatry Reports* 15(3): 347.

Wong, C. (2002) Post-traumatic stress disorder: advances in psychoneuroimmunology. *Psychiatry Clinics of North America* 25: 369–383.

Young, L. and Stoll, S. (2003) Proteins and amino acids. In L. E. Matarese and M. M. Gottschlich (eds), *Contemporary nutrition support practice* (2nd ed., pp. 94–104). New York: Saunders.

Young, S. N. (2007) Folate and depression: a neglected problem. *Journal of Psychiatry and Neuroscience* 32(2): 80–82.

7 ETHICAL PRACTICE AND DECISION-MAKING IN MENTAL HEALTH

JO AUGUSTUS

============================ LEARNING OBJECTIVES ============================

After studying this chapter you will be able to:

- consider the role of culture in decision-making;
- examine case examples associated with anti-discriminatory practices;
- describe the values associated with specific professional bodies;
- consider the models and theories that underpin decision-making processes.

INTRODUCTION

This chapter will introduce the complexities surrounding ethics in decision-making within mental health settings. Culture will be explored as an influential factor to effective decision-making, as well as associated theories and models. Hypothetical clinical cases will be presented to demonstrate both the challenges and opportunities that mental health professionals routinely face. Finally, consideration will also be given to diagnosis, choice of treatment interventions and the inequity of service provision.

Ethical practice both underpins and informs effective decision-making throughout mental health practices. From a bio-psycho-social perspective the following definitions apply (Cuthbert and Quallington 2008):

- Ethics are the moral principles that direct or guide an individual's behaviour.
- Decision-making is the cognitive processes that guide an individual to select a behaviour from different alternatives.

Therefore, in mental health practice, ethical decision-making is the moral principles that influence the steps we take in making choices when working with individuals. These decisions could involve discussions with the individual, their family or **carers** or happen separately as part of a **multidisciplinary team (MDT)**.

THE ROLE OF CULTURE IN ETHICAL PRACTICE

Ethical practice in **mental health** requires the application of the core conditions and an awareness of an individual's cultural background. Such an approach can facilitate an enabling and arguably more positive experience for the individual accessing mental health services and can also act as a model of good practice for the wider team including other mental health professionals. At an organisational level this can enable the effective delivery of service provision, through professionals and service users adopting a shared vision or collective identity. Ethical practices are closely linked to the cultural identity of both an individual and an organisation and adhering to such practices can ensure that mental health services are provided to individuals more equitably at a societal level. This links to cultural competence (see Chapter 10 for a more detailed discussion), which provides a way to demonstrate ethical principles: respect for persons; beneficence, e.g. doing good; non-maleficence, e.g. doing no harm; and justice, e.g. fair treatment of individuals. Therefore it is evident that ethical principles are an illustration of morals and values, formed by culture.

Tseng and Streltzer (2008) recognise the wider impacts of culture in mental health through the lens of cultural competence and in doing so highlight the importance of applying this lens to the individual's **recovery** goals. They identify three attributes:

1. *Cultural sensitivity*: an understanding of cultural diversity.
2. *Cultural knowledge*: an awareness of cultural diversity in the context of anthropology that could be obtained by gaining relevant experience.
3. *Cultural empathy*: an ability to connect on an emotional level with the cultural perspective.

A working knowledge of these attributes can be applied to interactions with individuals to understand the impact of culture. Cultural insight can also be used as part of clinical judgement, to ascertain if the mental health symptoms the individual is displaying are related to culture (Tseng and Streltzer 2008) and with such an awareness, an appropriate treatment can be suggested.

It is also important to acknowledge the culture of the mental health professional, as this may also play a role in decisions being made. When a mental health professional encounters an ethical dilemma, the decision made is, in part, influenced by their own culture and values, but may not reflect the values shared by the individual receiving treatment. In addition, current schools of thought underpinned by current research, may also influence decisions being made (Tseng 2004) and therefore, the individual service user, mental health professional, organisation and current research all play a role in shaping decisions made in ethical practice. Despite such components playing an influential role in decision-making processes, the individuals involved may largely be unaware of these, e.g. they are unconscious transactions. It is possible that such a lack of awareness can lead to discriminatory practices. Thus, consideration needs to be given to what support systems can be put in place to highlight awareness and aid ethical decision-making.

SHARED DECISION-MAKING

Shared decision-making is facilitated by two or more individuals who hold relevant expertise and collaborate in making complex decisions about patient care. Here, expertise is largely viewed as an individual's competence, including their skills and experience (Bradley and Green 2017). Such expertise can be from mental health professionals who hold an in-depth understanding of a particular issue, including risks and available interventions. Importantly relevant expertise is also often gained from the individual and may include their family and/or carer (Charles, Gafni and Whelan 1999). The key characteristics of shared decision-making could be seen as follows (adapted from Bradley and Green 2018):

- collaboration between at least the patient and professional;
- sharing of information and consideration of patient concerns;
- discussion of treatment options and patient choice;
- an agreement about decisions made, agreed and reviewed.

Shared decision-making is therefore a model of communication that facilitates an egalitarian approach (Bradley and Green 2018). There are a variety of personal and cultural values being shared as part of the decision-making process (Joosten et al. 2008). Arguably this is seen as a shift away from the traditional paternalistic approach where the decision is made for the client based on scientific inquiry. In promoting such autonomy there is a movement towards informed choice, broadening out from informed consent (Joosten et al. 2008).

There exists much research to support shared decision-making for both physical and mental health difficulties, where the consensus is an emphasis on **person-centred care**. Enabling individuals to make decisions about their particular long-term conditions or **severe and enduring mental health difficulties** has often demonstrated improved outcomes, e.g. rates of recovery or reduction of relapse. Ishii et al. (2014) found that individuals with a diagnosis of **schizophrenia** reported improved outcomes such as satisfaction about the interventions received. With improved satisfaction there is greater likelihood of adhering to care plans, which are indicators of long-term recovery (Gray, Robson and Berssington 2002; Vermeire et al. 2001).

In addition, beyond the metrics, all parties being involved can enhance the experience of mental health patients. The responsibility involved is shared, with an emphasis on the individual being responsible for their own recovery journey and thus supported to make choices (Bradley and Green 2018).

WHAT IS PERSON-CENTRED CARE?

Being person centred in mental health settings involves equipping the individual with the correct knowledge and enabling them to be actively involved with their care practice. This approach should be applied to all **service providers** at all stages of decision-making, from assessment to discharge planning. A therapeutic relationship between all those involved can facilitate specific aspects of care, such as in medication management, where issues that may arise around concordance can be managed more effectively (Charles et al. 1999; Junghan et al. 2007), thus enabling the individual to increase efficacy through directing decisions within the wider multi-disciplinary team. Therefore, shared decision-making is essential in order to take a bio-psycho-social approach to person-centred care.

Although the benefits of shared decision-making are evident, they are not applied consistently in mental health practice. It is recognised that individuals with a mental health diagnosis often request involvement in care planning, which may or may not be met (Adams, Drake and Wolford 2007; O'Neal et al. 2008). Equally, professionals are often criticised for not being collaborative, or for lack of involvement with the individual, their family or carers, which can lead to feelings of disempowerment (Anthony and Crawford 2000; Gray et al. 2009). This could relate to how individual professionals interpret and place value on to the importance of shared decision-making (Hamann et al. 2009; Seale et al. 2006). Therefore, there is a need to review how shared decision-making processes are applied in order to make patient-centred recommendations moving forward.

MENTAL HEALTH PROFESSIONALS

Having an awareness of anti-discriminatory practices is an essential component of decision-making and can help promote anti-oppressive practices. The personal cultural and social model (PCS) provides a framework to analyse the different levels of discrimination and oppression (Thompson 2006). Based on an approach developed by Dalrymple and Burke (1995), Thompson (2006) identified three levels: personal, cultural and social (see Figure 7.1).

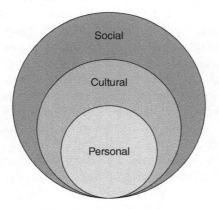

Figure 7.1 Personal, cultural, social model.

Source: Adapted from Thompson (2006).

In Thompson's (2006) three levels the personal refers to the individual's viewpoint, including their attitudes, beliefs, and interpersonal relationships. As shown in Figure 7.1, the personal is located within both the social and cultural areas of the model, as the individual's views are supported through the other two levels. The individual's culture determines rules that shape how the individual sees themselves, others and the world. This includes interactions that occur between others and the environment. The personal and cultural are located within the social area of the model. The social includes the order, rules and structures that operate in society.

An organisational example:

A new ward opens in an acute psychiatric hospital and job adverts for a new ward manager appear on the staff notice board.

Personal: A female mental health nurse comments to her male colleague that he should not apply for the job because English is not his first language.

Cultural: The local community centre next to the hospital holds the viewpoint that those who do not speak English as a first language should work in menial jobs that do not involve speaking to the public.

Societal: A national newspaper headlines focuses on individuals moving to the UK from aboard and taking all the health care jobs. This also highlights how patient care is compromised by 'foreigners' as care practices are seen as being different abroad. Legislation is being passed to prevent people working in the UK unless they meet certain criteria.

The above example highlights how the PCS model could be applied as a lens to specific examples. Here seemingly routine procedures within a hospital are influenced by different levels, resulting in discriminatory and oppressive practices. By applying the lens to different situations, discriminatory practices can potentially be highlighted and therefore help to change how processes are instigated.

The PCS model is applied to the social work discipline, however it is applicable to all professions, highlighting that anti-discriminatory and anti-oppressive practices occur at different levels and are embedded within each other. It is important to note that while change can occur at each level, challenge may be more difficult at some levels. For example, challenging discriminatory or oppressive practices at an individual or cultural level, such as an individual or individuals within an organisation. Here challenge and change can happen through following local processes, e.g. whistleblowing. However, applying this to larger groups in society could be more challenging. In practice mental health professionals can start this important process by reflecting on their own attitudes and beliefs as well as cultural and societal structures.

Reflection plays an important role in decision-making processes in ensuring they are conducted in line with specific ethical practices. This may include self-reflection, e.g. through keeping a diary, taking notes during clinical supervision or monthly supervision meetings. Such practices may be governed by professional bodies, although not all mental health professionals are required to do so (see Chapter 4 for identification of different professionals).

The PCS model aims to address discrimination that could occur in all the relationships between the professional and individual and the wider social context and in doing so challenge social disadvantage, including inequalities (Burke and Harrison 2009; Dominelli 2002). In order to put the PCS model into practice the next section will explore the anti-oppressive practice from the perspective of a social worker.

CAREERS IN FOCUS: SOCIAL WORK

Social workers maintain professional relationships and support individuals and families that may be experiencing difficulty. This may include ensuring that vulnerable individuals are safeguarded against harm. The role demands making difficult decisions, which may be against the wishes of those involved.

The PCS model enables the social worker to challenge discrimination through an awareness of the role of the self, the employer and the wider society and enable the individual(s) the social worker is working with to move away from inequality. For a social worker to effectively work in this way a level of self-awareness is required that facilitates an understanding of how they can enable or disable social injustices that could otherwise potentially result in discriminatory practices. Such self-awareness should include the social worker's own past experiences and an awareness of how this might affect their present practice. This includes how their role could be seen to exert power over an individual and the impact this can have as part of decision-making processes.

CASE STUDY 7.1: BREACHING CONFIDENTIALITY

(*This is a fictional case study*)

The situation

Gwynn is a social worker registered with the Health and Care Professions Council (HCPC) and has over 22 years' experience working with individuals with severe and enduring mental health difficulties, their families and carers. Currently she is working on a project funded by social services, to prevent individuals who have been previously detained under the Mental Health Act from being readmitted to hospital. Her office was moved twice in the last 8 months, including all her paperwork, and she now sits in an office next to the busy library and a community cafe. It is a busy area with various groups and classes running throughout the day, evenings and weekends. She only uses one filing cabinet, which is an old fashioned unit and doesn't have a lock. Gwynn didn't feel it was important to lock the cabinet because she doesn't put very detailed information in the patient's case files and has a light caseload. This is an approach she has always taken. She feels this allows her to focus on being with the patient and focus on their needs. Gwynn works from 8.30 am until 5.30 pm, Monday to Friday and although she closes the door to her office, it is not locked, as the lock is broken. She spends most of her time in the office except when she makes home visits 2–3 times a month. Gwynn made a non-urgent request in writing for maintenance to fix the door lock and replace the filing cabinet once, three months ago. Around 5 weeks ago after the Easter bank holiday weekend, her line manager, who works in another office, arranged an urgent meeting with her.

The member of the public's perspective

Gwynn's manager described how a member of the public had reported seeing a number of current patient files marked private and confidential with her name on. The files

(Continued)

(Continued)

contained personal information about patients' histories including mental health diagnoses and criminal convictions. The member of the public became very upset as he felt they might pose a risk to his community. He had entered the office mistakenly trying to find a register for the group he was covering that evening. The filing cabinet was a mess and it is possible he had seen many of the files. Gwynn's manager asked her to explain how a member of the public had access to this information.

The social worker's perspective

Gwynn expressed her anger that he should not have gone into her office and that he should be reported to the police. She then became defensive, stating that it wasn't her fault that she had had to move offices twice and she had done all she could to ask for a door lock. Gwynn then detailed that many of the patients had a form of **dementia** and some had died since the project began three years ago and also that she was acting in a patient-centred way. Finally, Gwynn reminded her manager of her 6-month absence from work and how she felt she wasn't supported on her return 8 months ago.

The outcome

Gwynn's manager suspended her from work, pending an investigation. The findings from this investigation were referred to Gwynn's regulatory body, the HCPC, for further scrutiny. The findings were presented at an HCPC disciplinary panel, where Gwynn presented her perspective supported by her union representative. The panel found that Gwynn had been in breach of confidentiality. The panel also felt that Gwynn's explanations were poor and she had been dismissive of the seriousness of her oversights about storing information about patients in her care. In addition, it was noted that she discriminated against those patients with dementia and those who had since died, disregarding them, their family and carers as having experienced no impact following breach of confidentiality. They decided that her membership of HCPC would be suspended for a period of 12 months, after which time it would be reinstated. Gwynn's employer also suspended her for 12 months and referred her to undertake a course on data protection and ethical practice, prior to returning to work and that on her return she would need to shadow and be shadowed by a senior colleague for up to 12 months. The patients, families and carers were all informed of the breach and no further action was taken.

Points to consider

Consider what might have influenced Gwynn's decision-making processes and explain why she acted in this way. This may include her past constructs about the importance of some aspects of her work, e.g. considering her approach as being shaped by what she had always done. What may have stopped her considering the impact of her actions on others? Finally, what learning must now happen to prevent this happening again? Using the PCS model is helpful to understand the different elements of oppression and discriminatory practice, as follows.

PCS model applied: Gwynn's perspective

Personal: I don't think it's important to keep detailed notes, I'd rather spend time with the clients I am working with. From my perspective this is patient-centred care.

Cultural: The organisation has always done things this way, they expect me to do more and they are slow to respond to my requests.

Social: The media reported three times last week that health professionals don't spend enough time with clients.

Do you think this is direct or indirect discrimination?

Gwynn's actions could be seen to directly discriminate against individuals in her care, with a diagnosis of dementia, which is considered a protective characteristic under the **Equality Act (2010)**. Dementia is a progressive condition and therefore is considered as a physical and mental impairment (Equality Act 2010). Therefore, the individuals discriminated against in this example could make a formal or informal complaint. This may involve gaining specialist advice from an independent organisation.

The role of direct or indirect discrimination needs to be explored in order to facilitate anti-oppressive and anti-discriminatory practices. Dominelli (2002, p. 15) looks at this in the context of three levels:

1. *Intellectual*: to understand the ways of working in a way that enables anti-oppression.
2. *Emotional*: the capacity to confidently deal with discrimination and oppression and to constantly reflect on one's practices in order to continually develop.
3. *Practical*: to apply the ideologies of anti-oppressive practices.

Thompson's (2006) PCS model was both designed for and has influenced social worker practices by gaining the recognition of how individuals are affected by personal, cultural and societal structures that interact and influence how individuals operate in the social world. It is therefore recognised that social workers need to go beyond simply understanding and move towards applying their knowledge in order to challenge discrimination.

Ethics plays an important role in decision-making between the individual and professional. Some decisions can be subtler, however, but can have a big impact on the care being provided.

CAREERS IN FOCUS: PSYCHOTHERAPY/COUNSELLING

Psychotherapy aims to support an individual to resolve difficulties they may be encountering, as a result of past or present issues. Different modalities of counselling place emphasis on difficult aspects of therapeutic change. However, there is a general consensus that change happens through therapeutic alliances created between the **counsellor** and individual. This role requires consideration of the ethical consequences and also the impact on the therapeutic relationship (Lehr and Sumarah 2004; Neukrug, Lovell and Parker 1996). Therefore, decisions made need to be done from a multidimensional perspective that accounts for all those involved.

CASE STUDY 7.2: ETHICAL DILEMMA IN RECEIVING GIFTS

(*This is a fictional case study*)

The situation

Pete qualified as a psychotherapist over 5 years ago, having been made redundant from a company he worked for as a human resources manager for over 20 years. He works in a busy community health centre that provides both individual and group-based interventions for individuals with symptoms of mild to moderate **anxiety** and **depression**. In the last 8 months Pete has noticed an increase in the severity of the mental health difficulties of the individuals he is working with. This is something he meant to discuss with his clinical supervisor, however he hasn't had the time. Pete's manager asked him and colleagues to increase the number of clients he has been seeing for a fixed term only, to help manage the waiting list. Pete has a strong work ethic and agreed with his manager to provide an evening clinic once a week. Pete began working with a client called Katie, a lady in her late thirties who had been referred to the service with symptoms of depression following the break-up of her relationship. During the first few sessions they discussed her relationship difficulties as an adult in the context of poor parenting and her experience of being adopted. Katie attended the evening clinic and prior to a session they had to wait outside the office for a meeting to finish that had overrun. Katie noticed there were flowers and chocolates in the nearby kitchen area and commented on them. Pete stated they were a gift from a former patient. Katie had completed 6 months of weekly sessions and commented that she had been feeling much better for longer periods of time. Katie arrived for her next appointment with a gift for Pete to thank him. The gift was a gold-coloured pen inscribed with his name and looked expensive. Pete thanked Katie and explained that he could not accept the gift as it was against the practice policy. Pete also made this judgement based on his experience as an HR manager. Katie became very upset in the session and left early. Two weeks later Pete's manager made an appointment with him to discuss a complaint letter he had received from Katie.

The client/Katie's perspective

Katie had written a detailed account of her session with Pete; this included her thoughts and feelings about her most recent session. This made reference to the conversation when Pete highlighted to Katie the gift he received from another patient and she couldn't understand why he couldn't therefore accept her gift. She described becoming more frustrated that he kept referring to the policy. Katie also provided detail that Pete should have understood how not accepting the gift had triggered bad memories from her past and subsequently has led to her symptoms deteriorating. Although she doesn't want to speak with Pete, Katie agreed to speak with Pete's manager and discuss this further.

The supervisee/Pete's perspective

Pete was confident in his decision that he had followed local policy not to accept any gifts from clients. In particular that the gift was very personal, as it had his inscribed name on it. He felt that accepting the gift would be crossing a boundary between his professional and personal life. He had discussed this with Katie at length, using all his counselling skills, however he was aware that as she was so upset in session she may not have heard everything he was saying. Katie posed many questions and Pete answered them with reference to policy, although he didn't know how to answer the question about accepting the gift from the other patient. Katie decided to leave the session early, which Pete acknowledged and completed a risk assessment. Pete found himself ruminating about this session and arranged to speak to his supervisor the next day.

The outcome

Pete and his manager met to discuss the session and feedback he had gained from meeting with Katie. They discussed at length what happened, what could have been done differently and what has been learned that could be taken forward. First, they discussed how Pete had accepted a gift from another client because he could share it with the whole team. By contrast, he couldn't share the pen as it was too personal. It appeared that Pete had been too focused on policy and had thus not realised the impact this would have on the client. Also, he realised how he had also become preoccupied with the meaning of accepting the gift from a psychodynamic perspective. He also reflected that because he was so fixed in his thinking he may have appeared to be aggressive in tone with the client. Finally, he realised now how an earlier casual conversation with Katie may have also had implications. It was agreed with his manager that Pete would invite Katie to a meeting with them to discuss a way forward. Pete would meet with his supervisor more frequently to discuss this and as part of his appraisal consider attending further training courses.

Points to consider

The above example highlights that there is often more than one approach that can be taken when making a decision. A guiding principle could be that of making decisions that have an evidence base. While the steps needed to take an evidence-based approach are not always clear, the decisions should be made in a consistent and ethical way. For example, the following steps could be considered when making decisions:

1. Refer to the professional codes of practice, e.g. the BACP, HCPC, BABCP.
2. Refer to organisational policies, e.g. safeguarding.
3. Refer to national guidance and law, e.g. the Bribery Act 2010.
4. Seek supervision, e.g. from a clinical supervisor or manager.
5. Contact the professional body via email or telephone.
6. Undertake self-reflection using a reflective model, e.g. a diary using Driscoll's (2007) 'what, so what, now what'.

A psychotherapist's values and past experiences are also influential and may be combined with ethical codes, embedded within professional bodies and organisations, enabling decisions to be made (Koocher and Keith-Spiegel 2008). Mandatory ethical practices form a

(Continued)

(Continued)

minimum expectation, whereas aspirational ethical practices arguably enable decisions to be made in the best interest of the client (Corey et al. 2015). If Pete had considered the impact of his actions, would he have taken a different course of action?

Using the PCS model is one way to help understand factors that influence decision-making processes:

PCS model applied: Pete's perspective

Personal: If I accept personal gifts then I am in breach of my employer and professional registration.

Cultural: The organisation only accepts some gifts from patients.

Social: The national news has reported how accepting gifts is seen as favouring one person against another and is often associated with bribery.

Ethical dilemmas in psychotherapy are often multifaceted as there are cultural, social and interpersonal elements to consider. Here the interpersonal factors relate to the therapeutic relationship between the client and therapist. For example, not accepting the gift may interrupt the alliance that has been built over a period of time, because the client feels rejected. Values play an important role in the decision-making processes; that may include integrity and the recognition that what happens in the therapy room may also happen in the client's daily life. Thus emphasising the importance of modelling good practices as part of the session, including professional relationships. If the therapeutic alliance is affected, then the session can be used to manage the client reactions differently. For example, encouraging the client to notice if they often feel rejected in day-to-day life and considering alternative ways to respond to this and learning to respond differently to such reactions and manage emotions in line with the client's values. It is important to note that there are no prescriptive steps in ethical practices and decision-making, rather there exist guiding frameworks. Although it should be acknowledged that self-reflection is an essential component for all professionals within health care settings to ensure that collaborative ethical decisions are made.

PROFESSIONAL VALUES AND PRINCIPLES TO GUIDE ETHICAL DECISION-MAKING

By definition values are seen as being complex and multifaceted, however, they are integral to practices within mental health and influence or guide decisions being made (Cuthbert and Quallington 2008). A health care professional's values are shaped by their past and can be seen as a system of beliefs, principles or standards held by an individual. This may include judgements about what they regard as important. The meaning of values may vary depending on the context, such as the value of a particular item, e.g. a house; belief system, e.g. political ideation; emotion, e.g. empathy; and morals, e.g. sense of what is right or wrong (Pattison 2004). In the context of mental health, values are the beliefs, principles or standards that professionals hold and that influence their interactions with others around them (Cuthbert and Quallington 2008).

It is also recognised that within certain helping professions, the professional's own values may influence the therapeutic relationship. Therefore, the professional should manage these so they do not influence the client (Corey et al. 2015; Houser, Wilczenski and Ham 2006). This is most commonly associated within psychotherapy disciplines, although arguably it features in many other professions. For example, in psychotherapy, managing counter-transference within a session can minimise the impact a therapist's values have on the client (Corey et al. 2015; Francis and Dugger 2014). Although it should be noted that an entirely 'value-free' session may be difficult to achieve, as the processes may be unknown or unconscious. However, the therapist's willingness to explore these processes in supervision or their own personal therapy may help to minimise the impact they may have (Kocet and Herlihy 2014).

WHAT IS TRANSFERENCE AND COUNTERTRANSFERENCE?

Transference is described as displacement by the individual of feelings from the past, in particular with relation to their parents, on to the figure of the therapist. **Countertransference** denotes the unconscious emotional reactions the therapist has towards the individual they are working with (Feltham, Hanley and Winter 2017).

Where the therapist's values have not been managed, the client may inadvertently be at risk of harm. For example, if the therapist's values significantly differ, the therapist may choose not to engage with the client or refer them elsewhere (Ford and Hendrick 2003; Shiles 2009). This could lead to the client having to undertake further assessments, longer waiting times and ultimately discourage the client from engaging in therapy.

Professional codes of practice provide a collection of shared values: a guiding framework that mental health professionals are expected to adhere to and maintain, such as 'do no harm' (Betan 1997; Corey et al. 2015; Francis and Dugger 2014). Many professional bodies hold similar values as shown in Table 7.1.

As shown in Table 7.1, professionals could be accredited by, registered with or simply belong to a professional body, although not all professionals are associated with a professional body, which can present challenges to some organisations or those working independently. It is disputed that if professionals are not associated with a professional body they could pose a risk to the individuals they work with. However, risk or bad practice can still occur and equally can lead to disciplinary proceedings and the individual losing their professional status (Herlihy, Hermann and Greden 2014). Ultimately the employer decides if the job requires professional registration, unless the individual works independently, e.g. as a psychotherapist.

Table 7.1 Values associated with professional bodies

Health and Care Professions Council (HCPC)	GMC (General Medical Council)	The British Association for Behavioural and Cognitive Psychotherapies (BABCP)	The British Association for Counselling and Psychotherapy (BACP)
Transparency	Excellence – we are committed to excellence in everything that we do	Act in the best interests of service users	Respect human rights and dignity
			Alleviate symptoms of personal distress and suffering
			Enhance people's well-being and capabilities
Collaboration	Fairness – we treat everyone fairly	Maintain high standards of assessment and practice	Improve the quality of relationships between people
			Enhance the quality of professional knowledge and its application
			Strive for the fair and adequate provision of services
Responsiveness	Transparency – we are honest and strive to be open and transparent	Respect the confidentiality of service users	Facilitate a sense of self that is meaningful to the person(s) concerned within their personal and cultural context
			Appreciate the variety of human experience and culture
Value for money	Collaboration – we are a listening and learning organisation	Keep high standards of personal conduct	Increase personal resilience and effectiveness
			Protect the safety of clients
			Ensure the integrity of practitioner–client relationships

Models and theories that underpin decision-making processes

There are various theories and models that can be used by mental health professionals to support thought processes surrounding decision-making. There are various models to consider and that are applicable to different settings. For example, a mental health nurse working in an inpatient acute psychiatric unit will most likely use a different approach to a psychotherapist working in a community-based health centre (Case et al. 2008). The following is not an exhaustive list, however it provides an overview of the three models available for mental health professionals to use.

Practice-based model

Practice-based models are practical in application rather than being theoretically based. This approach provides a series of stages that can be used as part of the decision-making processes. Corey et al. (2015) propose one such model, providing eight stages from the identification of a difficulty to ethical consideration and discussions with multidisciplinary team, all feeding into a final decision. While this approach provides a logical framework for a **practitioner** to apply, it also promotes confidence in decision-making and a clear rationale. Limitations of such an approach lie in its process-driven nature, which may not enable the level of personalisation needed to facilitate person-centred care. In addition, while a wealth of information is accrued, this could be overwhelming for an individual using this approach.

Social constructivist model

Social constructivism is a school of thought embedded in sociological theory of knowledge, where 'reality' is seen as being constructed through interpersonal interaction. Therefore, knowledge is gained through connections with other people and is socially constructed (Cottone 2001). In the context of decision-making, the social constructivist model views the decision as being made through exchanges between two or more individuals, e.g. counsellor and client or care coordinator and service user. Here, the professional does not lead and thus decisions are made collaboratively, arguably in a transparent manner. However, it would be expected that the professional implements the decisions made. Negotiations may be used where differences occur and agreement is not reached; it is important this happens as a shared language so all parties are understood. In addition, where disagreement occurs, stages could be taken to resolve these, such as seeking guidance from other professionals to gain consensus. This is an ongoing process of discussion and where relevant should include wider mental health professionals.

A transcultural integrative model

This model seeks to integrate and apply different decision-making models, including the social constructivist model (Cottone 2001; Garcia et al. 2003). The model integrates multicultural theory that encourages the use of a culture or society as a frame of reference. In doing so it recognises that different cultural communities hold their own strengths and weaknesses and thus is relational by its approach. The model adopts a step-by-step approach in a linear format. Interestingly it also encourages professionals to take a reflective approach as well as accounting for cultural difference, collaboration between different professionals and the individual engaging with a service provider, adopting an integrative perspective. Therefore, in doing so it adopts an ecological approach that considers factors from the individual, their relationships and influential factors at a societal and community level. Taking such a collaborative approach ultimately seeks to work towards an ethical decision (Garcia et al. 2003).

Theories that underpin decision-making processes

There are various ethical theories in existence that can help professionals make decisions in mental health. Theories provide a systematic means of understanding a situation that may occur in practice. Beauchamp and Childress (2013) outline key theories relevant to making ethical decisions that can be applied to a variety of different settings:

> *Consequentialism*: from an ethical perspective, consequentialism stipulates that the correct moral response is associated with an outcome or effect of a particular action taken.

> *Deontology*: places respect on the individual, emphasising the value of the individual rather than the outcome of an action. Its focuses on rules, responsibilities and duties in the context of being ethical.

> *Principlism*: integrates different ethical theories that are consistent with individual, societal or cultural belief systems. There are four key ethical principles: autonomy, beneficence, non-maleficence and justice.

> *Virtue ethics*: highlights the moral character of the individual, such as those seen in professional regulatory bodies, e.g. the HCPC.

The above theories offer shared principles that focus on the individual and aim to act in the best interest of the individual and in doing so safeguard the individual from harm. The 'do no harm' principle dates back to Hippocrates or the Hippocratic oath and is embedded in professional regulatory bodies. Failure to recognise decisions in the best interest of an individual could lead to complaints or disciplinary action being taken. This could be seen to operate on a continuum from what might be regarded as minor to serious situations relating to poor boundaries. There are also lesser-discussed research areas relating to the well-being of the professional, which is recognised as 'burnout'. Here the professional may not be aware of their **psychological well-being** needs and this could impact on the decisions they make in mental health practice. Here self-reflection is imperative, along with access to regular structured clinical supervision in order to mitigate such risks. While such risks cannot be prevented, decision-making theories and models can help minimise the risk of unethical decisions being made.

CONCLUSION

This chapter has explored some of the issues mental health professionals may encounter when working with individuals. It has sought to introduce some key theories and models along with examples from practice. It is recognised that over time a mental health practitioner will develop higher-order thought processes as part of their decision-making. Such development involves clinical supervision, continual self-reflexivity and professional development and ongoing experience. The role of professional bodies is not only to regulate professionals, but also to be responsive to societal change. Such cultural competence seeks to improve the assessment and treatment of individuals that encounter service providers.

REFERENCES

Adams, J. R., Drake, R. E. and Wolford, G. L. (2007) Shared decision-making preferences of people with severe mental illness. *Psychiatric Services* 58: 1219–1221.

Anthony, P. and Crawford, P. (2000) Service user involvement in care planning: the mental health nurse's perspective. *Journal of Psychiatric Mental Health Nursing* 7: 425–434.

Beauchamp, T. L. and Childress, J. F. (2013) *Principles of biomedical ethics* (7th ed.). New York: Oxford University Press.

Betan, E. J. (1997) Toward a hermeneutic model of ethical decision making in clinical practice. *Ethics and Behavior* 7(4): 347–365.

Bradley, E. and Green, D. (2018) Involved, inputting or informing: 'shared' decision-making in adult mental health care. *Health Expectations* 21: 192–200.

Burke, B. and Harrison, P. (2009) Anti-oppressive approaches. In R. Adams, L. Dominelli and M. Payne (eds), *Critical practice in social work* (2nd ed.). Basingstoke, UK: Palgrave Macmillan.

Case, J. C., Plaisance, P. M., Renfrow, J. J. and Olivier, B. N. (2008) Playing with a 'full DECK': a creative application of the integrative decision-making framework of ethical behavior. *Rehabilitation Education* 22(3–4): 171–184.

Charles, C., Gafni, A. and Whelan, T. (1999) Decision-making in the physician–patient encounter: revisiting the shared treatment decision-making model. *Social Science and Medicine* 49: 651–661.

Corey, G., Corey, M. S., Corey, C. and Callanan, P. (2015) *Issues and ethics in the helping professions* (9th ed.). Stamford, CT: Brooks/Cole.

Cottone, R. R. (2001) A social constructivism model of ethical decision-making in counseling. *Journal of Counseling and Development* 79(1): 39–45.

Cuthbert, S. and Quallington, J. (2008) *Values for care practice*. Exeter: Reflect Press.

Dalrymple, J. and Burke, B. (1995) *Anti oppressive practice social care and the law*. Maidenhead, UK: Open University Press.

Dominelli, L. (2002) *Anti oppressive social work*. Basingstoke, UK: Palgrave Macmillan.

Driscoll, J. (2007) *Practising clinical supervision: a reflective approach for healthcare professionals* (2nd ed.). Edinburgh: Bailliere Tindall Elsevier.

Equality Act (2010) c.15. www.legislation.gov.uk/ukpga/2010/15/contents (accessed 16 February 2016).

Feltham, C., Hanley, T. and Winter, L. A. (2017) *The SAGE handbook of counselling and psychotherapy* (4th ed.). Los Angeles, CA: Sage.

Ford, M. P. and Hendrick, S. S. (2003) Therapists' sexual values for self and clients: implications for practice and training. *Professional Psychology: Research and Practice* 34: 80–87.

Francis, P. C. and Dugger, S. M. (2014) Professionalism, ethics, and value-based conflicts in counseling: an introduction to the special section. *Journal of Counseling and Development* 92: 131–134.

Garcia, J. G., Cartwright, B., Winston, S. M. and Borzuchowska, B. (2003) A transcultural integrative model for ethical decision making in counseling. *Journal of Counseling and Development* 81(3): 268–277.

Gray, B., Robinson, C., Seddon, D. and Roberts, A. (2009) An emotive subject: insights from social, voluntary and healthcare professionals into the feelings of family carers for people with mental health problems. *Health and Social Care in the Community* 17: 125–132.

Gray, R., Robson, D. and Berssington, D. (2002) Medication management for people with a diagnosis of schizophrenia. *Nursing Times* 98: 38–40.

Hamann, J., Mendel, R., Cohen, R., Heres, S., Ziegler, M., Buhner, M. and Kissling, W. (2009) Self-reported use of shared decision-making among psychiatrists in the treatment of schizophrenia: influence of patient characteristics and decision topics. *Psychiatric Services* 60: 1107–1112.

Herlihy, B. J., Hermann, M. A. and Greden, L. R. (2014) Legal and ethical implications of using religious beliefs as the basis for refusing to counsel certain clients. *Journal of Counseling and Development* 92(2): 148–153.

Houser, R., Wilczenski, F. L. and Ham, M. (2006) *Culturally relevant ethical decision-making in counseling.* London: Sage.

Ishii, M., Okumara, Y., Sugiyama, N., Hasegawa, H., Noda, T., Hirayasu, Y. and Ito, H. (2014) Efficacy of SDM on treatment satisfaction for patients with first admission schizophrenia: study protocol for a randomised controlled trial. *BMC Psychiatry* 14: 111.

Joosten, E. A., DeFuentes-Merillas, L., de Weert, G. H., Sensky, T., van der Staak, C. P. and de Jong, C. A. (2008) Systematic review of the effects of shared decision-making on patient satisfaction, treatment adherence and health status. *Psychotherapy Psychosomatics* 77: 219–226.

Junghan, U. M., Leese, M., Priebe, S. and Slade, M. (2007) Staff and patient perspectives on unmet need and therapeutic alliance in community mental health services. *British Journal of Psychiatry* 191: 543–547.

Kocet, M. M. and Herlihy, B. J. (2014) Addressing value-based conflicts within the counseling relationship: a decision-making model. *Journal of Counseling and Development* 92: 180–186.

Koocher, G. P. and Keith-Spiegel, P. (2008) *Ethics in psychology and the mental health professions: standards and cases* (3rd ed.). New York: Oxford University Press.

Lehr, R. and Sumarah, J. (2004) Professional judgement in ethical decision-making: dialogue and relationship. *Canadian Journal of Counseling* 38(1): 14–24.

Neukrug, E., Lovell, C. and Parker, R. J. (1996) Employing ethical codes and decision-making models: a developmental process. *Counseling and Values* 40(2): 98–106.

O'Neal, E. L., Adams, J. R., McHugo, G. J., Van Citters, A. D., Drake, R. E. and Bartels, S. J. (2008) Preferences of older, middle-aged and younger adults with severe mental illness for involvement in shared decision making in medical and psychiatric settings. *American Journal of Geriatric Psychiatry* 16: 826–833.

Pattison, S. (2004) Understanding values. In S. Pattison and R. Pill (eds), *Values in professional practice: lessons for health, social care and other professionals.* Oxford: Radcliffe Medical Press.

Seale, C., Chaplin, R., Lelliott, P. and Quirk, A. (2006) Sharing decisions in consultations involving anti-psychotic medication: a qualitative study of psychiatrists' experiences. *Social Science and Medicine* 62: 2861–2873.

Shiles, M. (2009) Discriminatory referrals: uncovering a potential ethical dilemma facing practitioners. *Ethics and Behavior* 19: 142–155.

Thompson, N. (2006) *Anti-discriminatory practice* (4th ed.). Basingstoke, UK: Palgrave Macmillan.

Tseng, W. S. (2004) Culture and psychotherapy: Asian perspectives. *Journal of Mental Health* 13: 151–161.

Tseng, W. S. and Streltzer, J. (2008) *Cultural competence in health care.* New York: Springer.

Vermeire, E., Hearnshaw, H., Van Royen, P. and Denekeris, J. (2001) Patient adherence to treatment. *Journal of Clinical Pharmacy and Therapeutics* 26: 331–342.

8 EQUALITY AND DIVERSITY IN MENTAL HEALTH PRACTICE

JO AUGUSTUS

=========================== LEARNING OBJECTIVES ===========================

After studying this chapter you will be able to:

- understand what equality and diversity means in mental health settings;
- understand laws relevant to equality and diversity;
- consider the different types of discrimination that occur in **mental health**;
- explore the impact of discrimination;
- consider ways to promote anti-discriminatory practices.

INTRODUCTION

Equality and diversity is fundamental to mental health practice. Ensuring that both access and service provision is equitable and fair is an essential component of any mental health service and should be integral to its design, rather than additional. Individual difference should be accounted for and identified barriers overcome as part of **person-centred care**. Therefore, the provision of services treats individuals as equal, prompting dignity and respect.

It is essential for professionals to have an understanding of equality and diversity in order for it to be implemented effectively at an organisational level. This chapter defines equality as 'ensuring individuals engaging in a service have equal access irrespective of their background, capabilities or lifestyle'. Diversity is 'the recognition of and respect of individual difference that may include systems of beliefs, culture or values'. Discrimination can occur when an individual is treated unfairly because of their differences.

This chapter will outline the legislative frameworks, explore what discrimination is and how it may occur and consider the impact of discrimination in mental health settings. Finally, ways to challenge mental health discrimination will be briefly discussed.

The current context

The World Health Organisation (WHO) recognises the fundamental rights of everyone without distinction to enjoy a high standard of health (WHO 2003). However, nationally and internationally there remains significant inequality in access to health care, including physical and mental health services. Owen and Khalil (2007) relate this to **service providers** failing to prioritise issues surrounding diversity until very recently. This is the case, even though socio-economic changes and multiculturalism have put pressure on services to meet the changing demands of a diverse society. Here diversity relates to the acknowledgement and value of difference and equality creates fairness where all can participate and have an opportunity to achieve their potential. NHS England (2018) stipulated that difference has to be both valued and recognised in order for there to be equality of opportunity. The WHO (2003) views diversity as practices of anti-discrimination in the context of one's own human rights. They detail individual components of what constitutes diversity, such as religion, national or social origin or sexual orientation and health status including diagnosis of HIV or AIDS.

Within the UK the equality agenda has often focused on accessible and responsive service providers (Department of Health and Social Care 2018). In doing so, ensuring that public services are open to all within the diverse communities that they are based. Partnership working forms a large part of promoting equality and challenging discrimination. This facilitates person-centred service provision where services are led by the individuals accessing them (Owen and Khalil 2007). Therefore, socially inclusive agendas need to be continuously reviewing the effectiveness of their approaches to equality and diversity.

LEGISLATION

The purpose of legislation is to set out a framework of rights and responsibilities by which the country is governed. In the UK, the government uses its lawmaking powers to pass legislation in the form of Acts of Parliament. Examples include the Mental Capacity Act 2005 or the **Equality Act 2010**. Sometimes Parliament delegates its lawmaking powers to other government departments, particularly where only a minor change to the law is needed. This is referred to as secondary legislation and leads to the formation of regulations and statutory codes of practice. As an example, in 2012 the coalition government used secondary legislation to amend the list of banned substances contained within the Misuse of Drugs Act 1971, in response to growing concerns about new psychoactive substances (also known as 'legal highs').

In the UK, Parliament has legislative supremacy, meaning that the laws it makes must be followed by the courts (Blakemore and Greene 2004). However, the higher courts still have a role in lawmaking in that the cases they decide shape the interpretation of legislation.

In relation to equality, legislation has an impact on the provision of services, both directly through equalities legislation and indirectly through the regulation of service providers. It also regulates the employment relationships that exist within care settings. An understanding of the legislative background is therefore essential to an understanding of equality and diversity. The legal context of mental health law is explored in more detail in Chapter 2.

Legislation, sometimes called statutory law, is a law made by a governing body to regulate. This may also authorise, grant or restrict. In the context of events, legislation defines the governing legal principles that outline the responsibilities for providers such as local authorities, in order to safeguard the public. Please see Chapter 2 for a more detailed account of mental health law. In the context of equality and diversity there are four key laws relevant to those working in mental health settings. These are outlined below.

The Mental Capacity Act 2005

The purpose of the Mental Capacity Act was to make new provisions in law relating to people who lack **capacity** (to make decisions for themselves). It also set up the Court of Protection, a new court with responsibility for making financial and welfare decisions for those people who cannot make those decisions for themselves.

It aimed to enhance protection:

- by encouraging individuals, where possible, to make decisions for themselves and providing an adaptable framework for those that lack capacity to make decisions themselves, which acts to put the individual at the centre of decision-making processes;
- by empowering individuals to plan ahead to the future when they may lack capacity.

The Equality Act 2010

The Equality Act 2010 came into force on 1 October 2010. Its primary purpose was to combine and simplify over 100 other separate pieces of equality legislation that existed at the time of the Act. This Act provides the legal framework for equality, both in relation to employment and to the provision of services. The Equality Act sets out both the 'protected characteristics' that are protected in law, and the kinds of discrimination from which protection exists. There are nine protected characteristics set out in the Equality Act 2010: age, disability, gender reassignment, marriage and civil partnership, pregnancy and maternity, race, religion or belief, sex and sexual orientation. It is worth noting that while many other forms of discrimination may exist, it is only these nine characteristics that are formally protected in UK law.

WHAT DOES THE PHRASE VULNERABLE ADULTS MEAN?

Vulnerable adults include individuals who are unable to protect themselves from harm or take adequate care of themselves. Vulnerability could be related to age, disability or physical illness.

The Human Rights Act 1998

The Human Rights Act 1998 came into force in October 2000 to 'guarantee the rights and freedoms' set out in the European Convention on Human Rights and incorporate them into UK law (Human Rights Act 1998). An explanation of the detailed operation of the Human Rights Act 1998 is beyond the scope of this book but it is worth noting that it sets out a number of high-level principles that may impact on the mental health agenda, including:

Article 5: The right to liberty and security.

Article 8: The right to respect for private and family life.

Article 9: Freedom of thought, conscious and religion.

The Care Act 2014

The Care Act 2014 came into effect in April 2015 and its aim was to reform 'the care and support for adults and the law relating to the support for carers'. It details the duties local authorities have in relation to establishing the eligibility of an individual's needs for publicly funded care provision. Under the Care Act this includes carrying out assessments and access to independent advocacy.

DISCRIMINATION AND STIGMA

Discrimination is often seen as actions, practices and processes that prevent the equal treatment of or disadvantage individuals from a particular social grouping or categorisation in society (Cooper and Dunn 2009). Therefore, discrimination is behaviour deemed biased and giving unfair advantage to a group in society. **Stigma** can be seen as a judgement or opinion held by individuals or groups of individuals within society and if acted on they could be seen as being discriminatory (Bryne 2000). Thus stigma is seen as characterised by attitudes associated with disparage, which separates out individuals from one another. This can include processes of individuals being wrongly blamed or disgraced (Cooper and Dunn 2009). In doing so, such actions may harm or deprive another social grouping (Dovidio et al. 2011). Attitudes are often influential aspects within discriminatory practices. Here attitude refers to an organisation of beliefs, emotions and actions directed to a specific area in society (Hogg and Vaughan 2005). In the context of mental health this could result from societal attitudes that view psychopathology as a risk, difficult or burdensome. Such attitudes can direct stigma and discrimination towards individuals displaying symptoms associated with mental health. González-Torres et al. (2007) noted that much of the stigma and discrimination relates to prejudice specific to labelling individuals as exhibiting deviant, lazy or dangerous behaviour. This could lead to these individuals being excluded from social groups, such as those within the workplace.

Allport (1954) recognised that favouring ingroups is influential in intergroup relations, which may operate at the expense of others. This encompasses bias in both attitudes and resource allocation, which does not necessarily include derogation (Brewer 1999). However, it is important to note that research has not focused on favouring the ingroup and outgroup derogation (Brewer 1999; Dovidio et al. 2011). A link could be made between ingroup favouritism and the expression of behaviour towards the outgroup, e.g. aggression (Dovidio et al. 2011). The intensity of the attitude or emotion expressed by the ingroup could also relate to the level of discrimination towards an outgroup (Brewer 1999). For example, avoiding a particular social group could be viewed as mild discrimination. This can often be seen in reports both nationally and internationally surrounding conflict, such as the reported genocide of the Rohingya who are a Muslim ethnic minority (Ibrahim 2018). While recognising the intensity of discrimination, this shouldn't be used to undermine the impact, but it can be useful to highlight awareness of discrimination.

Different types of discrimination

What is direct discrimination?

Direct discrimination is the legal term that applies if an individual is treated less favourably than someone else because of a protected characteristic. It may be lawful to require job holders to have particular characteristics (known as genuine occupational requirements), e.g. being a male **carer** may be a genuine occupational requirement in an inpatient residential unit that only has male residents. However, these exceptions are rare (Equality Act 2010).

Example

Paul explained to a group of his colleagues that he was diagnosed with **depression** after his mum died two years ago. He is a bank health care assistant. He overheard the ward manager say that she needs reliable staff and will avoid giving him shifts because he is likely to take sick leave due to his depression.

What is indirect discrimination?

Indirect discrimination is the legal term that is used to describe situations where an organisation implements policy or procedure or makes decisions that on the surface appear to promote equality, however, in reality they lead to individuals being treated less favourably because of a protected characteristic. Indirect discrimination may be less obvious, however, can impact individuals in the same way as direct discrimination. There is, however, an exception as indirect discrimination may be justified where it is a 'proportionate means of achieving a legitimate aim' (Equality Act 2010, s.19(2)(d)). This is known as objective justification. Objective justifications cannot be used to justify direct discrimination (with the exception of direct discrimination because of age) (Equality Act 2010).

Example

Samira's place of work is a care facility where she has worked for over 8 years, which has recently undergone a restructuring. During a meeting her new manager told her she is no longer allowed to cover her face when working with clients. Samira is an observant Muslim and wears a full face covering.

However, Samira's employer may be able to justify this action. A legitimate aim may be to ensure that clients can see her facial expressions as part of developing a therapeutic alliance. However, it would only be proportionate to require Samira to remove her face covering when she is actually working with clients and not at other times.

What is harassment?

Harassment is 'unwanted conduct related to protected characteristics', which has the purpose or effect of 'violating [a person's] dignity or creating an intimidating, hostile, degrading, humiliating or offensive environment for [them]' (Equality Act 2010 s.26(1)).

What is victimisation?

Victimisation is where a person is treated less favourably because they have asserted rights or have given evidence in relation to discrimination, as defined by the Equality Act 2010.

Types of discrimination in mental health practice

Different types of discrimination exist that are relevant to mental health practice; some are explicit while others are more subtle. Mental health stigma can broadly be separated into two categories, social stigma and self-stigma, also known as perceived stigma. Here social stigma is typified by harmful attitudes and behaviour towards an individual with difficulties associated with mental health, resulting from the label of the mental health diagnosis (Dovidio et al. 2011; Rössler 2016; Scheff 1966). By contrast, self-stigma is a term frequently used to denote the processes in which an individual with a mental health difficulty internalises the stigma. This can have a significant impact on feelings of shame that impact on their **recovery**, e.g. outcome of treatment (Rössler 2016). Bradley and Green (2018) highlight another type of stigma termed courtesy stigma, which denotes the impact that stigma has on the people connected to the individual with a physical or mental health difficulty that is stigmatised. This is an under-researched area and given the potentially distressing impact this could have, further research is warranted.

Unconscious bias, sometimes known as implicit bias, recognises that we all tend to make decisions based on assumptions that stem from our cultural, educational background and personal experiences. Decision-making can be instantaneous and we may not even be aware of the types of bias that are influencing our decisions. This means that when we engage in decision-making we tend to treat more favourably others who are similar to ourselves in terms of background, gender, race, ethnicity and other protected characteristics (Bonomo 2016; Cuellar 2017). Microaggressions link to unconscious bias in that the aggressor may not be aware of their actions. Microaggression occurs where minority groups are subjected to low-level aggressive behaviour by members of the dominant cultural group (Sue 2010). Infantilisation is used to describe treating an adult like a child, such as by a carer or health care assistant to a patient (Link and Phelan 2001). This process may be unconscious and with the carer or health care assistant acting with the patient's best interest in mind. However, this can lead to marginalisation and denial of an individual's personhood (Agmon, Sa'ar and Araten-Bergman 2016; González-Torres et al. 2007).

Haslam and Dovidio (2010) explored four specific components that could be seen to promote and maintain discriminatory practices. These are personality and individual differences, group conflict, social categorisation and social identity. They are examined in more detail below.

There are various theoretical approaches taken to understand the characteristics of personality and individual differences. The use of scapegoating as an outlet for frustration can be a framework used to understand causation. For example, oppression of the Jews during the Holocaust. The stereotype content model perspective recognised that minority groups in society that are deemed successful are more liable to be scapegoated (Glick 2005). Social dominance theory can be used to understand individual difference and how intergroup bias may exist between groups (Dovidio et al. 2011).

In early attempts to understand discrimination, bias that existed in society was seen as abnormal. However, this developed into an understanding that biases can characterise large groups. Therefore, the concept of group conflict developed to enable a focus on functional relations between different groups. Theories surrounding this concept, such as realistic group conflict theory, suggest that competition for resource at a group level can lead to measures being taken to restrict access to other groups (Scheff 1966).

Allport (1954) sought to recognise discrimination as being part of everyday society rather than something that is abnormal. Allport (1954) proposed the notion that discrimination results from social categorisation or an individual's desire to classify themselves as belonging to a group, thus excluding themselves from another group. Here the processes surrounding social categorisation create the foundations for social bias (Dovidio et al. 2011).

Social identity is the individual's awareness of their identity based on the group they belong to. Here social identify theory and self-categorisation theory can be used to understand intergroup behaviour, formed by personal and social identity. When social identity is embedded in a group the individual may view themselves as a collective and thus social bias may appear within a group (Onorato and Turner 2001; Tajfel and Turner 1979).

It is important to acknowledge that discrimination and stigma involve complex processes, however they can be understood through exploration of specific components. This is essential for discrimination to be challenged and for services to be more equitable in their provision. The next section will explore equality and diversity from a multidimensional perspective, focusing on specific characteristics of service users.

The impact of discrimination on mental health

Research indicates that discrimination is associated with an increasing risk of depression (Bhui et al. 2005; Perez-Garin, Molero and Bos 2016; Wallace, Nazroo and Becares 2016). Putting it simply, the act of discrimination could create an increasing sense of hopelessness, which is characteristic of depression. Unfair actions, such as insults, might relate to someone's sense of self or identity and marginalise an individual. This includes, however is not limited to, perpetrator and victim, because this could limit the awareness of discrimination to those who are discriminated against. As such the individual may develop feelings of worthlessness, vulnerability and worry about the future. It is important to acknowledge that such discriminatory practices can occur at any stage of the life course and in a variety of different environments.

The example in Case Study 8.1 highlights the impact on carer Julie, of what could be seen as the unfair treatment of her elderly mum.

CASE STUDY 8.1: JULIE – CARER PERSPECTIVE

Having been a carer for my mum over a number of years, I found our journey frustrating and emotionally draining. My mum had COPD [chronic obstructive pulmonary disease], which necessitated several hospital admissions and it was clear that after a few, no proper assessments of mum's needs were undertaken. Instead, because they thought she lived with me permanently I would turn up for a visit and find her belongings packed up on the bed ready for discharge. The ward staff did not bother to check with me. Eventually I had to insist that assessments were undertaken as mum developed **dementia** and wasn't safe to live on her own. Finally the promoting independence team became involved and liaised with me initially. At last! I thought! Assessments and social care would now be involved. After only a week I received a phone call to be advised that they were pulling out and had arranged for a care company to take over and a social worker would carry out an assessment. On the day of the prearranged visit, the social worker phoned to cancel, as it was his last working day for the authority. I resisted the cancellation and a reluctant social worker turned up and did an assessment. Some respite care was agreed, financial forms completed and the social worker advised that his senior would be holding the case until it was reallocated. Weeks went by without any contact. I phoned the senior who advised that mum was not eligible for respite as she had a family. I found that bad practice was systemic. The day after mum's funeral I received a letter from adult social care advising us that they were closing the case but if her condition worsened then we should notify them.

The notion of personhood can be eroded, arguably disabling the provision of person-centred care and treatment plans can shift towards staff-centred approaches (Agmon et al. 2016; González-Torres et al. 2007). At its extreme this can result in concerns specific to safeguarding. However, it is evident that the concept of discrimination can also inspire mental health professionals, as the example in Case Study 8.2 indicates.

CASE STUDY 8.2: PETER – REFLECTIONS ON MENTAL HEALTH AS A SOCIAL WORKER (SEE CASE STUDY 1.2 IN CHAPTER 1 FOR THE FULL VERSION)

As an undergraduate, I became interested in theories of institutionalisation, particularly Goffman's work on asylums in the United States and Townsend's work on old people's homes in the UK. These works haunted me as I began a career as a social worker and became 'part of the system' that continued to place individuals in large-scale institutions, without any thought for personalisation.

Although Bhui (2016) recognises that discrimination is not accepted as a cause of mental health or physical health difficulty, it is evident that unfair actions can result in symptoms that relate to **psychological well-being**. For example, in response to recurrent trauma of discrimination an individual may develop maladaptive coping strategies that are then adopted by existing social groups or continued by future generations (Infurna et al. 2016; McKenzie and Bhui 2007). However, such symptoms can be conceptualised as being characterised by mental health and therefore the acts of discrimination can be missed as the cause. This reinforces the need for all health care professionals to be aware of anti-discriminatory practices.

Interestingly, there is a growing body of research that recognises that from adverse experience individuals develop post-traumatic growth. In doing so individuals develop resilience that they continue to apply to new experiences. Thus, applying this to discrimination the individual is likely to learn about themselves and differences that exist between themselves and others (Bhui 2016). Such new constructs create an opportunity for different understanding and growth in anti-discriminatory practices. Any example lies in the British exit from the European Union (BREXIT) and attitudes towards fear of immigration leading to an increase in crime and/or overcrowding (Bhui 2016; Bhui et al. 2005).

Race

A race is a grouping of individuals based on shared physical or social qualities, viewed as fundamentally distinct by society (Caliendo and McIlwain 2010; Sue 2010). There exist various theories and research relating to gaining an understanding of harmful attitudes relating to racism and discrimination (Bhui 2016). Racist acts may include reference to skin colour or they may take a subtler form, such as stereotypes that surround arranged marriage as depicted in films. Periods of socio-economic change, such as BREXIT, appear to relate in part to hostility towards migrants resulting from the perception that migrants pose a threat to British citizens. Acts of racial discrimination could be seen as part of the sense of unhappiness relating to poor economic growth, e.g. low interest rates.

Ethnicity

Ethnicity is the state of belonging to a particular social group that has a shared national or cultural tradition (Caliendo and McIlwain 2010). Black and minority ethnic (BME) communities are recognised as often experiencing poorer health outcomes, which may include difficulties associated with accessing services (Owen and Khalil 2007). Over time there have been various initiatives implemented to overcome known barriers to engagement with mental health service provision. This included in part challenging the negative perception that services were unhelpful and involving the BME community in service developments (Bhui 2016). There was also a drive towards organisations working towards non-discriminatory practices through a workforce that has an awareness of equality and diversity. Services were encouraged to integrate provisions that are accessible to all rather than encourage segregation and in doing so provide a foundation for services to be person centred rather than problem focused.

Gender

Gender is a term applied to the complex arrangements between men and women, which incorporates reproduction, division of labour and the cultural aspects of masculine and feminine (Bradley 2013). There exists much debate about its meaning and the fluidity of its application to different contexts, which acts to intensify the contested nature of its definition (Glover and Kaplan 2000). Gender equality refers to fairness and justice in the distribution of resource allocation and allocation of responsibility between men and women (Bradley 2013). Gender inequality denotes unequal treatment on the basis of gender, originating from societal, cultural or global perspectives, for example (Glover and Kaplan 2000). It is an established school of thought that socio-economic status relates to access to resources, which in turn leads to disparities in both psychological and physical well-being (Link and Phelan 1995). Historically, the World Health Organisation recognised that gender differences need to be addressed at all levels of policy, including its development and implementation (WHO 2003). Traditionally the focus is on promoting women's physical and mental health, through the recognition that women hold less power than men and thus access to fewer resources. Also, the perception that acts of violence (e.g. rape) towards women exerted from men result from women's vulnerability (Vlachova and Biason 2005). However, it is important to acknowledge that gender-based violence affects both men and women. The quality standard produced by NICE (2016) addresses this through an acknowledgement of gender inclusivity in supporting individuals experiencing domestic violence and abuse. In contemporary society, where gender is a more fluid concept, future policy needs to be adapted to accommodate the needs of individuals beyond gender. Therefore, supporting a mental health workforce that can respond to the needs of the individual and are not constrained by the concept of gender.

Religion

There exists much debate over how religion is defined, in particular schools of thought surrounding what characterises being religious and non-religious. For the purpose of this discussion, definitions of religion can be considered from two perspectives: substantive and functional. Substantive refers to the key characteristics of religion, grounded in belief of phenomenon that is beyond human comprehension. Functional definitions relate to the effects of religion at an individual and societal level and may include its utility (Furseth and Repstad 2007). There is a link between psychological well-being and religious beliefs, which could relate to a sense of belonging or hope. Thus, if discrimination occurs on the basis of religion then it is likely to have an impact on an individual's mental health. Jordanova et al. (2015) highlight the lack of research into the impact of religious discrimination on mental health. However, research that has been conducted shows emerging evidence of an increase in prevalence of common mental health difficulties in those who experienced discrimination on the grounds of religion (Jordanova et al. 2015).

CASE STUDY 8.3: HARAM FOOD

Aala, a 20-year-old female observant Muslim, was admitted as an informal patient to an inpatient psychiatric ward following a diagnosis of anorexia nervosa that could not be managed in the community. This appeared to be the first episode for her and was thought to have been triggered by discussions of marriage. Aala presented as being non-verbal and at times unresponsive to any external stimulus, although this varied. She did on occasion say yes or no very quietly, however, never gave any eye contact. A meal plan was agreed with her psychiatrist within two hours of her admission, although Aala did not consent. As part of her meal plan Aala was to be given a choice of food from a pictorial menu, which she sometimes engaged with, although it often caused her distress. Her family did not attend her admission as they lived over 150 miles away and therefore, visited infrequently.

Three weeks into her stay, the ward was understaffed over the summer bank holiday weekend and a health care assistant decided to select Aala's food to save her distress and also to save time. She felt she had a good working alliance with Aala and approached her with kindness. Aala ate some of the food presented to her at dinner time, although she became particularly distressed at times, which staff supported her with. While it was noted the intensity of distress was unusual for Aala, they labelled this as being typical of an eating disorder diagnosis.

A few days later Aala's family complained to the hospital director that Aala had been given Haram food, which is food forbidden by Muslims. On discussion with her family it emerged that English was not her first language and Aala did not understand until she had eaten much of the food and realised it was Haram from its consistency and taste. Aala's family also explained that she had once witnessed her friends and tutors being killed by terrorists at her school. She had survived by hiding for over 24 hours before being found. When it was reported that she had survived, threats were made to her and her family. Her father applied for and was granted asylum when Asla was 5 years old. The incident at the hospital was reported to the CQC.

Consider the following questions:

What is the consequence of labelling being applied to Aala's response as 'being typical of an eating disorder'?

What key communication skills might you use?

How could this incident have been avoided?

What would you do to improve practice?

Hint: consider what information might be missed if staff focus solely on the mental health problem.

As Case Study 8.3 highlights, it is essential that care planning captures information about the whole person, from their religion to their history. This will minimise mistakes being made and allow the **multidisciplinary team** to work in a person-centred way that promotes collaboration and autonomy. Arguably these are essential aspects of recovery.

Impact on family and carers

Carers can be defined as those who care for a family member, friend or someone who cannot cope independently and therefore needs help due to disability, frailty, illness or a mental health problem. The care they give is unpaid. The Care Act 2014 introduced an assessment and eligibility procedure between the carer and local authority. This enables the support needs of the carer to be addressed. Although the focus of research and consideration centres on the primary caregiver, it is important to acknowledge the contribution of the wider family, friends and community. It is approximated that there are 1.5 million individuals caring for those with a diagnosis of dementia and/or mental health difficulties (Bradley and Green 2018). Those individuals who continued to be cared for at home save the economy a significant amount of money. However, despite this caregivers often face social isolation and have access to few resources.

The shift of care provision from inpatient settings to the community has put increasing pressure on carers to provide care, whether this is for short-term or long-term rehabilitation. There is, however, often a lack of preparedness for the provision of such care for individuals with mental health problems. As a result, carers could experience difficulties in their own psychological well-being and this can impact negatively on other aspects of their lives, such as financial problems, social isolation or poor physical health (Jeyagurunathan et al. 2017). Research has found that the incidence of mental health difficulties in caregivers doubles when compared to the general population (El-Tantawy, Raya and Zaki 2010; Oldridge and Hughes 1992). Although the incidence varies depending on the severity of the mental health problem, e.g. whether the individual being cared for has a common mental health problem or **severe and enduring mental health illness**. Carer burden is therefore increasingly being recognised as an important agenda item for policy makers.

WHAT IS CARER BURDEN?

Carer burden can be described as the stress experienced by the caregiver as a result of caring for an individual with support needs (LoboPrabhu, Molinari and Lomax 2008).

Academics have often explored the carer burden from a multidimensional perspective, for example, Lawton et al. (1989) suggested five dimensions:

- subjective burden;
- impact of caregiving;
- mastery;
- satisfaction; and
- reappraisal.

This approach considers stressors that the individual copes with from resources they have already developed or by accessing resources in their external environment. Therefore, the caregiver's psychological well-being is seen as the outcome of caring. Here social resources are an important component of how the caregiver views their role as a carer.

Another approach proposed by Lawton et al. (1991) is the two-factor model that considers the well-being components for the caregiver as well as the stress that it can cause. In other words, the first factor of the model denotes that the caregiver can experience positive affirmations from the care they provide, which could be from the individual or wider community. Whereas the second factor recognises that the demands of caring can deplete the caregiver's resources impacting negatively on their physical and psychological well-being.

These approaches have been criticised for their lack of relevance for those caring for those across the life course, as the model was produced from research that focused on care of older adults, and also for the simplistic approach of cause and effect, which neglects to consider the holistic aspect of caregiving. However, this approach provides a framework that highlights the support needs of carers with the aim of reducing carers' burden (LoboPrabhu et al. 2008).

Carer burden can be measured in a number of different ways, including the use of outcome measures that are used in everyday practice to screen, monitor and measure the severity of symptoms. Some outcome measures are free to use while others incur a fee, thus it is important to check this before using. For example, Jeyagurunathan et al. (2017) used the following measures:

- The World Health Organisation Quality of Life instrument assessed the quality of life of the caregiver (WHOQOL Group 1998). It features 26 items and produces scores for four domains: physical health, psychological, social relationships and environment. This measure also includes overall quality of life and general health.
- The General Anxiety Disorder (GAD-7) and Patient Health Questionnaire (PHQ-9) scales were used to measure psychological well-being (Spitzer et al. 2006). GAD-7 features seven items that the user rates on a scale, focusing on features of generalised anxiety disorder. PHQ-9 features nine items that again the user rates on a scale of how often they have been experiencing signs of depression (Kroenke and Spitzer 2002).
- The Family Interview Schedule (FIS) features 14 questions assessing the impact of caregiving that relates to financial, social, interpersonal and work-related difficulties (Sartorius and Janca 1996).

Coomber and King (2013) acknowledge that carer burden research is often on cross-sectional studies, rather than longitudinal research. In other words, research is more often conducted at one moment in time as opposed to over a long period of time, although cross-sectional research can provide valuable information from a population or subset population at a given point in time. For example:

Jeyagurunathan et al. (2017) researched the psychological well-being and quality of life for carers of individuals with different diagnoses ranging from psychosis, anxiety disorders and also those with dementia. The results highlight the significant impact caring can have on the caregiver's quality of life and psychological well-being. Therefore stressing the need for carers to receive psycho-social support including education programmes.

Coomber and King (2013) researched the carer burden that resulted from caring for individuals with an eating disorder diagnosis. The findings from this showed that the caregiver often experiences high levels of burden and emotional distress.

The longitudinal research also looked at predictors of carer burden and found a correlation with maladaptive coping strategies. For example, the carer blaming themselves, avoiding or disengaging with the person they are caring for and/or rejecting the diagnosis. Similar to Jeyagurunathan et al. (2017), although more specific, Coomber and King's (2013) research findings focused on specific interventions to support carers in managing their emotional distress and developing ways to address carer need.

Bradley and Green's (2018) research highlights that staff are developing an awareness of the need for shared decision-making with family members of individuals with serious mental illness (SMI). This could include inviting family members to multidisciplinary meetings to create a shared sense of recovery for that individual. The research showed that staff act as gatekeepers to involving family and that moving forward there needs to be a focus on family as part of the recovery processes. Akin to Jeyagurunathan et al.'s (2017) research, there needs to be a training programme for effective shared decision-making. Interestingly, Bradley and Green (2018) also indicate there is a role for peers as part of recovery.

González-Torres et al.'s (2007) research hypothesised that individuals with a diagnosis of **schizophrenia** are most likely to experience stigma, which may act as a barrier to recovery. The findings indicate that such discrimination led to social isolation and self-stigmatisation, which reinforced a sense of difference between themselves and others. This also impacted on the family by leading to social isolation and maladaptive coping strategies such as being over-protective. This could lead to unintended consequences of the individual developing an over-reliance on family, thus lack independence and increasing the carer burden. Interestingly they presented an example in northern Spain that introduced a community mental health centre, which arguably tackles stigma at a cultural and societal level (Thompson 2016). See Chapter 10 for further international perspectives on mental health.

It is evident from the above discussion that the impact of caring for someone with a mental health difficulty is vast. However, it is evident that there are certain themes such as carer burden that lead to psychological and/or physical health difficulties. Here historical maladaptive coping strategies are noted as predictors of carer burden. It is also apparent that stigma associated with mental health affects the way carers respond to the individual they are caring for, leading to over-reliance and delayed recovery. There is a recognition that shared decision-making with family members could help manage carer burden. Social isolation is a key feature where family and carers become distant due to prejudice and/or self-stigmatisation. Collectively it is evident that further support for carers is needed, whether this is through provision of a training intervention or peer support and research can then be conducted into its effectiveness and propose a model of carer well-being.

Challenging discriminatory practices

Anti-discriminatory practices have featured in service developments for many years, acting to ensure they are meeting the needs of the individuals using the services they provide. There is also a recognition that equality and diversity is a complex area, however it is one that needs to be addressed in order to provide equitable services that are consistently patient centred (Owen and Khalil 2007). Despite this Owen and Khalil (2007) have identified reports showing deficits in service provision to discriminated groups of individuals. While national policy seeks to provide equitable services, often service providers face challenges when trying to implement them (SCMH 2002). Owen and Khalil (2007) proposed a fourfold approach to overcome the identified challenges, which encourages awareness of the following:

1. The UK government has provided a framework to promote and enable equality and diversity agendas as part of public health. Public Health England has set equality objectives for 2017–2020 (PHE 2017). This outlines a phased development plan that includes stakeholders to promote a workforce that is diversity informed and in turn delivers equitable and fair services.
2. Historically there was a recognition that organisational cultures need to change in order to support a sustainable health service. Part of the focus was specific to mainstreaming. The NHS in England responded to the Equality Act 2010 by outlining specific equality duties (NHS 2017). This report adopts a values-based approach to providing high-quality care through developing equality and reducing health inequality. There is also an emphasis on partnership working and collaboration to advance practice.
3. The provision of educational programmes that aim to develop a culturally competent workforce (Campinha-Bacote 2002; Geron 2002; Nardi, Waite and Killian 2012). Such a model of training encompasses cultural awareness and knowledge delivered through experiential learning. This approach depends on the professional understanding the cultural identity of the individual they are working with.
4. Individuals should be approached from a holistic perspective, shifting away from labelling that could restrict practice (Owen and Khalil 2007) and thereby enabling person-centred care to be provided from the bio-psycho-social approach as needed.

Arguably challenging stigma and discrimination is an ongoing process that seeks to involve the personal, societal and cultural as integral drivers of change (Thompson 2016). Although this chapter has focused on the UK, good practice has been introduced from international examples. See Chapter 10 for more details about international mental health.

Experts by experience

It is also of great importance to involve experts by experience in both evaluating and developing mental health services. By definition experts by experience are individuals who have experienced themselves or care for others who have had difficulties associated with mental or physical health. There is also a recognition of co-production where both the expert by experience and the professional hold equal power and responsibility to make decisions (Mayer and McKenzie 2017). There is extensive research that attests to the value of experts by experience, in particular engaging marginalised groups in a positive way (Clark, Brudney and Jang 2013; Smith, Gallagher and Wosu 2012). Yet it appears that experts by experience are not consistently engaged in service development, thus there exists an opportunity to research the reasons for this.

CONCLUSION

It is essential that mental health professionals working in all settings uphold equality and diversity practices. There is clear legislative guidance and national policy designed to promote best practice. However, it is evident that such approaches are not consistently implemented in practice, which creates the risk of restricting access to service provision. However, there is much evidence of cultural change within organisations and drivers towards community engagement, which provide models of good practice that can be universally adopted. In an increasingly globalised world it will be expected that mental health professionals have an appreciation of equality and diversity in order to provide effective person-centred care.

REFLECTIVE EXERCISE 8.1

In order to assess how well diversity is managed, consider the setting you work in, including the individuals accessing the service and ask yourself the following questions:

1. What protected characteristics as outlined in the Equality Act 2010 do the individuals that access the service have? How is this information obtained?
2. How does the service respond to the identified needs of the individual?
3. How does your workplace ensure that everyone has equal access to services?
4. What impact does this have on care provision?
5. Is there anything else that can be done to develop the service?

REFERENCES

Agmon, M., Sar'ar, A. and Araten-Bergman, T. (2016) The person in the disabled body: a perspective on culture and personhood from the margins. *International Journal for Equity in Health* 15: 147.

Allport, G. W. (1954) *The nature of prejudice.* Cambridge, MA: Addison-Wesley.

Bhui, K. (2016) Discrimination, poor mental health, and mental illness. *International Review of Psychiatry* 28(4): 411–414.

Bhui, K., Stansfeld, S., McKenzie, K., Karlsen, S., Nazroo, J. and Weich, S. (2005) Racial/ethnic discrimination and common mental disorders among workers: findings from the EMPIRIC study of ethnic minority groups in the United Kingdom. *American Journal of Public Health* 95: 496–501.

Blakemore, T. and Greene, B. (2004) *Law for legal executives.* Oxford: Oxford University Press.

Bonomo, Y. (2016) Addressing unconscious bias for female clinical academics. *Internal Medicine Journal* 46(4): 391–391.

Bradley, E. and Green, D. (2018) Involved, inputting or informing: 'shared' decision making in adult mental health care. *Health Expectations* 21(1): 192–200.

Bradley, H. (2013) *Gender.* Cambridge: Polity Press.

Brewer, M. B. (1999) The psychology of prejudice: ingroup love or outgroup hate? *Journal of Social Issues* 55(3): 429.

Byrne, P. (2000) Stigma of mental illness and ways of diminishing it. *Advances in Psychiatric Treatment* 6(1): 65–72.

Caliendo, S. M. and McIlwain, C. D. (2010) *The Routledge companion to race and ethnicity.* London: Routledge.

Campinha-Bacote, J. (2002) The process of cultural competence in the delivery of healthcare services: a model of care. *Journal of Transcultural Nursing* 13(3): 181–184.

Clark, B. Y., Brudney, J. L. and Jang, S. G. (2013) Coproduction of government services and the new information technology: investigating the distributional biases. *Public Administration Review* 73(5): 687–701.

Coomber, K. and King, R. (2013) A longitudinal examination of burden and psychological distress in carers of people with an eating disorder. *Social Psychiatry and Psychiatric Epidemiology* 48(1): 163–178.

Cooper, V. and Dunn, B. (2009) *Understanding social work practice in mental health.* London: Sage.

Cuellar N. G. (2017) Unconscious bias: what is yours? *Journal of Transcultural Nursing* 28(4): 333–333.

Department of Health and Social Care (2018) Equality duty in 2017. https://assets. publishing.service.gov.uk/government/uploads/system/uploads/attachment_ data/file/708857/equality_duty_in_2017_dhsc.pdf (accessed 9 June 2018).

Dovidio, J. F., Hewstone, M., Glick, P. and Esses, V. M. (eds) (2011) *The SAGE handbook of prejudice, stereotyping and discrimination.* London: Sage.

El-Tantawy, A. M. A., Raya, Y. M. and Zaki, A. (2010) Depressive disorders among caregivers of schizophrenic patients in relation to burden of care and perceived stigma. *Current Psychiatric Therapies* 17: 15–25.

Equality Act (2010) c.15. www.legislation.gov.uk/ukpga/2010/15/contents (accessed 16 February 2016).

Furseth, I. and Repstad, P. (2007) An introduction to the sociology of religion: classical and contemporary perspectives. London: Routledge.

Geron, S. M. (2002) Cultural competency: how is it measured? Does it make a difference? *Generations* 26(3): 39–45.

Glick, P. (2005) Choice of scapegoats. In J. F. Dovidio, P. Glick and L. A. Rudman (eds), *On the nature of prejudice: 50 years after Allport* (pp. 244–261). Malden, MA: Blackwell Publishing.

Glover, D. and Kaplan, C. (2000) *Genders.* London: Routledge

González-Torres, M., Oraa, R., Arístegui, M., Fernández-Rivas, A., Guimon, J., González-Torres, M., Arístegui, M. and Fernández-Rivas, A. (2007) Stigma and discrimination towards people with schizophrenia and their family members: a qualitative study with focus groups. *Social Psychiatry and Psychiatric Epidemiology* 42(1): 14–23.

Haslam, S. A. and Dovidio, J. F. (2010) Prejudice. In J. M. Levine and M. A. Hogg (eds), *Encyclopedia of group processes and intergroup relations* (Vol. 2, pp. 655–660). Thousand Oaks, CA: Sage.

Hogg, M. and Vaughan, G. (2005) *Social psychology* (4th ed.). London: Prentice-Hall.

Human Rights Act (1998) c42. www.legislation.gov.uk/ukpga/1998/42 (accessed 16 February 2017).

Ibrahim, A. (2018) First they came for the Rohingya. *Foreign Policy* 228: 12–13.

Infurna, M. R., Brunner, R., Holz, B., Parzer, P., Giannone, F., Reichl, C. and Kaess, M. (2016) The specific role of childhood abuse, parental bonding, and family functioning in female adolescents with borderline personality disorder. *Journal of Personality Disorder* 30: 177–192.

Jeyagurunathan, A., Sagayadevan, V., Abdin, E., YunJue, Z., Chang, S., Shafie, S., Abdul Rahman, R., Vaingankar, J., Siow Ann, C., Subramaniam, M., Zhang, Y., Rahman, R. and Chong, S. (2017) Psychological status and quality of life among primary caregivers of individuals with mental illness: a hospital based study. *Health and Quality of Life Outcomes* 15: 1–14.

Jordanova, V., Crawford, M., McManus, S., Bebbington, P., Brugha, T. and Crawford, M. (2015) Religious discrimination and common mental disorders in England: a nationally representative population-based study. *Social Psychiatry and Psychiatric Epidemiology* 50(11): 1723–1729.

Kroenke, K. and Spitzer, R. L. (2002) The PHQ-9: a new depression diagnostic and severity measure. *Psychiatric Annals* 32: 1–7.

Lawton, M. P., Kleban, M. H., Moss, M., Rovine, M. and Glicksman A. (1989) Measuring caregiving appraisal. *Journals of Gerontology: Psychological Sciences* 44: P61–P71.

Lawton, M. P., Moss, M., Kleban, M. H., Glicksman, A. and Rovine, M. (1991) A two-factor model of caregiving appraisal and psychological well-being. *Journal of Gerontology: Psychological Sciences* 46: P181–P189.

Link, B. G. and Phelan, J. (1995) Social conditions as fundamental causes of disease. *Journal of Health and Social Behavior* (Special Issue): 80–94.

Link, B. G. and Phelan, J. C. (2001) Conceptualizing stigma. *Annual Review of Sociology* 27: 363–385

LoboPrabhu, S. M., Molinari, V. A. and Lomax, J. W. (eds) (2008) *Supporting the caregiver in dementia: a guide for health care professionals.* Baltimore, MD: Johns Hopkins University Press.

McKenzie, K. and Bhui, K. (2007) Institutional racism in mental health care. *British Medical Journal* 334: 649–650.

Mayer, C. and McKenzie, K. (2017) '... it shows that there's no limits': the psychological impact of co-production for experts by experience working in youth mental health. *Health and Social Care in the Community* 25(3): 1181–1189.

Nardi, D., Waite, R. and Killian, P. (2012) Establishing standards for culturally competent mental health care. *Journal of Psychosocial Nurse Mental Health Services* 50(7): 3–5.

National Institute for Health and Care Excellence (NICE) (2016) Domestic violence and abuse: quality standard 116. www.nice.org.uk/guidance/qs116 (accessed 19 September 2018).

NHS (2017) NHS England response to the specific equality duties of the Equality Act 2010: NHS England's equality objectives and equality information. www.england.nhs.uk/wp-content/uploads/2017/03/nhse-sed-response.pdf (accessed 7 May 2018).

NHS England (2018) NHS England response to the specific equality duties of the Equality Act 2010. www.england.nhs.uk/wp-content/uploads/2018/06/nhse-response-to-specific-equality-duties-of-the-equality-act-2010.pdf (accessed 5 October 2018).

Oldridge, M. and Hughes, I. (1992) Psychological well-being in families with a member suffering from schizophrenia: an investigation into long-standing problems. *British Journal of Psychiatry* 161: 249–251.

Onorato, R. S. and Turner, J. C. (2001) The 'I' the 'me' and the 'us': the psychological group and self-concept maintenance and change. In C. Sedikides and M. B. Brewer (eds), *Individual self, relational self, collective self* (pp. 147–170). New York: Psychology Press.

Owen, S. and Khalil, E. (2007) Addressing diversity in mental health care: a review of guidance documents. *International Journal of Nursing Studies* 44: 467–478.

Perez-Garin, D., Molero, F. and Bos, A. E. (2016) The effect of personal and group discrimination on the subjective well-being of people with mental illness: the role of internalized stigma and collective action intention. *Psychology Health and Medicine* 1–9.

Public Health England (PHE) (2017) *PHE equality objectives for 2017–2020.* https://assets.publishing.service.gov.uk/government/uploads/system/uploads/attachment_data/file/593090/PHE_Equality_objectives_2017_to_2020.pdf (accessed 7 May 2018).

Rössler, W. (2016) The stigma of mental disorders: a millennia-long history of social exclusion and prejudices. *EMBO Reports* 17(9): 1250–1253.

The Sainsbury Centre for Mental Health (SCMH) (2002) Breaking the circles of fear: a review of the relationship between mental health services and African and Caribbean communities. London: The Sainsbury Centre for Mental Health.

Sartorius, N. and Janca, A. (1996) Psychiatric assessment instruments developed by the World Health Organisation. *Social Psychiatry and Psychiatric Epidemiology* 31: 55–69.

Scheff, T. J. (1966) *Being mentally ill: a sociological theory*. New York: Aldine de Gruyter.

Smith, M., Gallagher, M. and Wosu, H. (2012) Engaging with involuntary service users in social work: findings from a knowledge exchange project. *British Journal of Social Work* 42(8): 1460–1477.

Spitzer, R. L., Kroenke, K., Williams, Janet B. W. and Löwe, B. (2006) A brief measure for assessing generalized anxiety disorder: the GAD-7. *Archives of Internal Medicine* 166(10): 1092–1097.

Sue, D. W. (2010) *Microaggressions in everyday life: race, gender, and sexual orientation*. Hoboken, NJ: John Wiley & Son.

Tajfel, H. and Turner, J. C. (1979) An integrative theory of inter-group conflict. In W. G. Austin and S. Worche (eds), *The social psychology of inter-group relations* (pp. 33–47). Monterey, CA: Brooks/Cole.

Thompson, N. (2016) *Anti-discriminatory practice* (6th ed.). Basingstoke, UK: Palgrave Macmillan.

Vlachova, M. and Biason, L. (2005) *Women in an insecure world: violence against women facts, figures and analysis*. Geneva: Geneva Centre for the Democratic Control of Armed Forces (DCAF).

Wallace, S., Nazroo, J. and Becares, L. (2016) Cumulative effect of racial discrimination on the mental health of ethnic minorities in the United Kingdom. *American Journal of Public Health* 106: 1294–1300.

The WHOQOL Group (1998) Development of the World Health Organization WHOQOL-BREF quality of life assessment. *Psychology Medicine* 8: 551–558.

World Health Organisation (WHO) (2003) *The world health report 2003: shaping the future*. Geneva: WHO.

9 SOCIETAL INFLUENCE ON MENTAL HEALTH

JO AUGUSTUS

═══════════════ LEARNING OBJECTIVES ═══════════════

After studying this chapter you will be able to:

- consider societal influences on the perception of **mental health**;
- describe the historical context of societal influence;
- understand barriers that may restrict access to **recovery**;
- understand theories and models that underpin **stigma** and discrimination.

INTRODUCTION

Societal influence is a term often used to describe the influence an individual or individuals can have on one another. For example, this could be a change in our belief system or behaviour as a result of an intentional or unintentional behavioural change of another individual. Such influence can have a profound impact on individuals accessing mental health services (Kawachi et al. 1997). As a culturally diverse society, mental health service provision has to be responsive to the social and cultural needs of its local population. Here culture is referred to as shared sets of beliefs and values between social groups (Hofstede 1991). Therefore, cultural and societal influence, are closely linked. It is important to note that culture is not the only factor to consider when trying to understand the issues surrounding access to services. It is evident that misinterpretation of culturally bound symptoms can impact on access to mental health services (Webber, Huxley and Harris 2011). Therefore, organisations need to be competent in the services they provide. However, in order to provide culturally competent services, there has to be an understanding of the influence of society and culture on mental health, which this chapter will explore (Kawachi et al. 1997).

THE CULTURE OF THE INDIVIDUAL AND THE PROFESSIONAL

Historical context

At the beginning of the nineteenth century, Western medicine recognised that the social aspects of an individual had an impact on disease, which arguably led to the advent of public health. The mid-nineteenth century saw the introduction of psychoanalysis as a way to treat mental health. The twentieth century brought an understanding that social and psychological components are of importance, in addition to the bio-medical (Porter 1997). There have been extensive developments in the provision of mental health services since the 1970s. In particular, the shift towards care provision in the community rather than inpatient settings and the awareness of cultural diversity (Shorter 1997). In addition, the publication of DSM-IV in 1994 gave more detailed references to cultural variation than earlier editions, encouraging a cultural formulation approach to be taken within the assessment (APA 1994). Although the bio-psycho-social model is subject to current criticism, it remains a helpful frame of reference (Engel 1980; Pilgrim 2011). Such an integration of approaches to the assessment and treatment of mental health enables a whole-person or holistic approach and provides the platform to meet specific cultural needs. See Chapter 1 for more detail on the history of mental health views, treatment and services.

The individual

It is widely recognised that culture is important, as this influences what the individual will identify with, within the context of the mental health setting. There may be symptoms that occur more frequently in some cultures and indeed the way those symptoms are communicated may differ. The meaning individuals give to the symptoms also plays an important role in the decision-making process of when, how and if they access services for support. In addition, culture may influence support networks, the development of coping mechanisms and any sense of stigma felt by individuals surrounding mental health. Symptoms may be discussed in different ways depending on the culture held, such as **depression** being described as a physical symptom (Lin and Cheung 1999). Thus, as consumers, the individual's culture is very present when accessing mental health services (Kleinman 1977).

It can be argued that cultures that are more noticeable in society are the ones that predominantly shape services. For example, Western medicine dominates the provision of physical and mental health services, based on the views of scientific **practitioners** and evidence-based models of care. In other words, knowledge acquired through scientific and empirical means. Although, through ever-evolving scientific enquiry, Western medicine is often viewed as a gold standard internationally (Hofstede 1991).

There are various interacting systems that influence the individual. Different systems theories exist in attempt to offer an understanding in order to support the individual. For example, Figure 9.1 looks at bioecological systems framework in the context of student mental health.

Barriers to accessing services

Ecological systems theory identifies five environmental systems that an individual interacts with (Bronfenbrenner 1979). This theoretical approach provides a structure to investigate the interactions an individual has within the community and wider society. In recognition of the importance of the individual, Bronfenbrenner developed the bioecological systems model that places the individual at the centre of the model (Bronfenbrenner and Morris 2006). Pinder-Amaker and Bell (2012) applied this model to explore student mental health crises in the context of the systems the students interact with (see Figure 9.1).

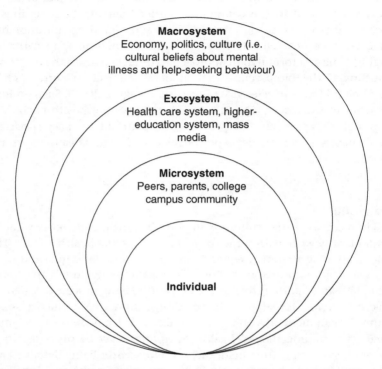

Figure 9.1 Bioecological systems framework for student mental health.

Source: Pinder-Amaker and Bell (2012)

Figure 9.1 shows the student (the individual) at the centre, surrounded by the microsystem that directly affects the student's mental health such as peers and the college campus community. The exosystem encompasses components such as the media and health systems, which are likely to influence peers and that in turn impact on the individual's mental health. The larger macrosystem includes societal beliefs about mental health. Here the bioecological approach is acknowledged to influence an individual's development and perception of mental health services, which could act as a barrier to accessing help. Through acknowledgement of such barriers, systems can be implemented to support the individual. The bioecological systems model can be applied to other individuals to improve the effectiveness of service delivery. DeVoe et al. (2018) applied the bioecological systems model to understand military service personnel with a diagnosis of post-traumatic stress disorder (PTSD) and the need for a family-based approach to provide effective support.

The mental health professional

It is equally important to recognise that mental health professionals hold their own culture, bound in the evidence base of their respective professions (Whaley 1998). Although professionals, bound by their registering bodies, maintain boundaries irrespective of their culture, it is inevitable that they bring their own culture to the therapeutic environment (Hunt 1995; Sue and Sue 1999). Research in the United States has shown this as being more apparent if the professional and individual are from different cultures (Wang, Berglund and Kessler 2000; Young et al. 2001). There is a risk here that information given is missed or minimised and the individual is therefore not understood (Whaley 1998). In addition, there may be different pre-conceptions about the role of the professional and individual, including the causes and treatment options. Such perceptions could lead to misunderstanding a diagnosis, which can have a significant impact on the individual, as Tish highlights in Case Study 9.1.

CASE STUDY 9.1: MORE THAN ONE DIAGNOSIS AND ITS IMPACT, TISH'S STORY

I was diagnosed as having depression, generalised anxiety disorder (GAD) and psychosis. The nature of the medication, prescribed by my psychiatrist, made any psychological intervention problematic as I was experiencing the effects of the 'chemical cosh' designed to deal with psychosis. I was also incapable of questioning this diagnosis even when evidence was uncovered suggesting that I was not experiencing psychotic episodes: the psychologist's view was that my supposed 'propensity for violence' had been taken out of context and was actually a 'fear of becoming violent', while the 'voices' I'd been hearing turned out to be very real with the discovery that my girlfriend *had* been in a relationship with the guy upstairs.

There were things that did work for me. The adoption of a little black cat stopped me from further attempts at suicide, got me out of bed every day and periodically got me out of my own front door. The gift of a bass guitar from a friend gave me an artistic output, eventually leading to more frequent adventures in the outside world when another friend invited me to participate in a band. The final part of my 'support system' was an invitation to get involved in an academic environment, with a service user and carer organisation, thus giving me an intellectual outlet. After coming off most of the medication, under the guidance of my GP, I was able to successfully engage with a psychologist and have now been free of medication for some time.

Here the cultural constructs held by the professionals may have influenced their decision-making as part of the assessment and treatment processes, but, arguably, diagnostic criteria do encourage the professional to appreciate differences in culture (Porter 1997).

ACCESS TO MENTAL HEALTH SERVICES

Cultural competency

Cultural competence sets out to identify the individual's culture and then construct knowledge, skills and policy (Bassey and Melluish 2013). Cross et al. (1989, p. 13) defined cultural competence as:

> a set of congruent behaviours, attitudes, and policies that come together in a system, agency, or among professionals and enable that system, agency, or those professionals to work effectively in cross-cultural situations. The word 'culture' is used because it implies the integrated pattern of human behaviour that includes thoughts, communications, actions, customs, beliefs, values, and institutions of a racial, ethnic, religious, or social group. The word competence is used because it implies having the capacity to function effectively.

Ultimately an awareness of cultural competence aims to provide safe and effective mental health services that are individualised to cultural needs. For effective delivery, mental health services have to develop a safe therapeutic environment, which relies on strong communication between the professional and the individual (Fuertes et al. 2006). Such an alliance relies on the professional's ability to understand the cultural identity that the individual presents. The development of new roles accessible within services, such as advocates, has responded to the need for cultural knowledge, including values, belief systems, language and customs. Such responsive services are recognised as culturally competent and have been developed in response to intrinsic need, rather than a scientific basis (Cross et al. 1989). Although research suggests that culturally competent services have encouraged patient outcomes and seen an improvement in symptoms and uptake of services (Bozarth 1998). However, much of this research has been conducted in the United States. Although there are similarities between the UK and the United States, it is important to recognise there are many socio-economic differences (Rathod et al. 2010).

Culturally competent services rely on organisations to provide services that are appropriate for the individuals accessing them (Bennett, Kalathil and Keating 2007; Bhui and Bhugra 2007; Department of Health 2003; Hall, Iwamasa and Smith 2003). This can present many challenges to **service providers** especially in the context of finances. Arguably with the creation of **Clinical Commissioning Groups (CCGs)** there is an opportunity for service providers to tailor their services to the specific need of the local population. However, if services are predominantly arranged at an organisational level they may be too far removed from the cultural needs and thus, not competent. This calls for individual involvement in order to provide consistent culturally competent services and a shift away from tokenism (Lo and Fung 2003; Tseng 2004), where tokenism attempts to create the impression of equality through superficial acts. Thus, shifting away from a top-down approach, the responsibility of cultural competence becomes a shared responsibility. Such shifts in service provision require research in order to develop evidence based on scientific enquiry (Bassey and Melluish 2013).

Social capital

The concept of social capital is often discussed in the context of well-being, in particular as a component of recovery. Here social capital is recognised as resources that are embedded within society that can lead to greater social mobility (Lin 2001). Such social capital is seen as being unequally distributed in society with access being particularly limited for those with **severe and enduring mental health difficulties** (Kawachi et al. 1997; Webber et al. 2011), which could be attributed to reduced social functioning due to the nature of their mental health difficulties, e.g. avoidance.

DIAGNOSIS AND CULTURE

Diagnosis is usually dependent on the mental health professional reporting in the following areas:

- an account of the type, intensity and duration of the presenting symptoms;
- direct observation of the individual's presenting problem and impact on functioning;
- clinical judgement about the symptoms, patterns and impairment of functioning that meet the diagnostic criteria.

Diagnosis of mental health difficulties often presents professionals with challenges. Largely this is due to the differences in the presenting problems that vary from person to person. The way such difficulties are communicated may also be misunderstood or described using unfamiliar references (Whaley 1998), as shown in Case Study 9.2.

CASE STUDY 9.2: SAI'S STORY

Sai is 34 years old. She moved from India to the UK 10 years ago after an arranged marriage and is a practising Hindu. She described settling quickly to her new environment, although missed her family and university friends. Following her third miscarriage she became easily agitated, angry and upset with her husband and her family. Her sleep deteriorated, she had reduced appetite and weight loss and began making mistakes at work, which led to her being suspended. She had visited her GP over 10 times in 3 months with abdominal pain for which there was no medical explanation. He prescribed her sleeping tablets and made her an appointment with the dietician to discuss meal planning.

Her husband made her an emergency appointment with the surgery after Sai reported increasing abdominal pain overnight. She saw a locum GP who happened to also be Indian. On examining Sai and looking at her case history the GP concluded that the phrase she used – 'headache in my stomach' – relates to her mood.

Question: What might be some of the difficulties here for Sai and the GP?

Hint: Consider cultural dietary differences and what a physical reference to mental health problems might mean?

Therefore, one of the key challenges in diagnosis is ensuring effective communication occurs between the individual and the mental health professional. Where appropriate, such communication may include the family and carer(s).

A diagnosis also derives from impairment of day-to-day functioning, however, a judgement is required as to whether this deviates from social norms. For example, auditory **hallucinations** are an accepted part of some cultures, but in other cultures it may constitute diagnostic criteria. Thus, a professional who is unaware of such cultural norms may make incorrect judgements. Expressions of distress can take different forms between cultures, for example somatisation, where distress may be described as a physical symptom. Justine highlights this in Case Study 9.3.

CASE STUDY 9.3: BODY MEMORY, JUSTINE'S STORY

I had 16 weeks of high-intensity CBT after being involved in a violent trauma many years before the physical symptoms of shaking and palpitations kicked in. I found the first four sessions of therapy very difficult as the therapist wanted to go over everything that had happened to me when I was attacked. I had tried to block this out of my memory so it was really hard to face it again after so long of avoiding it. I noticed that during and after these therapy sessions talking about what happened, I had a lot of physical pain, in fact it was the same pain as I had when I was originally assaulted. I found dealing with this physical pain on top of managing my symptoms and confronting the reality of what happened really trying and I almost stopped therapy at this point … the physical pain I experienced during and after therapy sessions seemed to mirror my injuries from the initial attack, so body memory was really significant. I know that's controversial but I experienced the pain all over again when going through what happened to me. I wish there was more acceptance of the reality of body memory for victims.

Table 9.1 shows some of the known differences between Eastern and Western cultures that need to be acknowledged in order to understand the impact they may have in everyday mental health care practices (Bassey and Melluish 2013). As such, cultural competence research has shifted away from practices to develop a professional's competence, to work with sociocultural factors that affect the individual (Bassey and Melluish 2013).

Table 9.1 Orientation differences between Eastern and Western cultures (adapted from Bassey and Melluish 2013)

Western cultures	Eastern cultures
Orientation	
Control	Acceptance
Personal autonomy	Harmony
Cognitivism	Emotionalism
Understanding by analysis	Understanding by awareness
Problem solving	Contemplation
Body–mind distinction	Body–mind–spirit unity
Individualism/privacy	Collectivism/group welfare
Mastery over nature	Harmony with nature

Future orientation	Past or present orientation
Free will	Determinism
Values	
Doing/activity	Being/fate
Time dominates	Personal interaction dominates
Human equality	Hierarchy/rank/status
Self-help	Birthright, inheritance
Competition	Cooperation
Directness/openness/honesty	Respect, restraint
Practicality/efficiency	Idealism
Materialism	Spiritualism
Informality	Formality

Although such discussions are beginning to be integrated into everyday clinical practice they are often criticised for being too limited to capture the complex and dynamic aspects of culture and mental health. Although it is important to recognise that such practices are constantly developing.

Stigma and discrimination

In the context of mental health, stigma is often seen as labelling an individual with undesirable attributes that are integral to their character, or that they may somehow be to blame for their difficulties (Upadhyay 2016).

REFLECTIVE EXERCISE 9.1

Leah left home aged 14 years after it emerged her mother's boyfriend had been abusing her. She lived in foster care for short periods and was then given a flat of her own three years later. Leah began to use unhelpful coping strategies to manage her emotions, such as deliberate self-harm, drug and alcohol use and restriction of food. She had been given various different mental health diagnoses from a young age, including low self-esteem, anorexia, anxiety and depression. It was also apparent that she had become involved in a series of abusive relationships with older men and on occasion the police became involved. Leah often presented at the accident and emergency department (A & E) in distress with wounds that needed stitching and she would often re-open the wound by pulling at the stitches. She became familiar to the medical staff on duty in A & E. On one occasion, Leah presented at A & E with her support worker with a deep cut to her upper thigh, which was bleeding profusely whenever she moved position. A member of the medical team approached her and stated that he was fed up with her coming to A & E and wasting their time. He suggested that she was doing this to herself deliberately for attention and that she would be seen by a member of the team only after the urgent cases had been treated. Leah became very distressed.

Question: What issues is Leah having to deal with that are specific to mental health stigma? What legislation may protect Leah?

Hint: Consider the culture of the individual and the professional.

Stigma typically leads to the formation of stereotypes and discrimination (Davidson, Stayner and Haglund 1998). As a consequence the individual may feel rejected from social groups and receive refusals from services they attempt to engage with, coupled with a sense of guilt and shame. Typically discrimination occurs at three different levels (Taylor and Dear 1981):

1. *Self-stigma*: occurs when the individual with a mental health diagnosis assumes the patterns of behaviour associated with the stereotypes that society imposes.
2. *Individual stigma*: negative behaviour shown towards individuals in the group that is assigned the stigma.
3. *Structural stigma*: discrimination that occurs inherently within societal structures, such as socio-economic policies.

Media influence

Ways of thinking about mental health are heavily influenced by constructs created around us, for example, a poster portraying the perfect body image (Dittmar 2008; Grabe, Ward and Hyde 2008; Groesz, Levine and Murnen 2002). Such constructs can be internalised and leave the individual with a negative view of themselves, imposed from the world around them (Ashikali and Dittmar 2012). In addition, there are particularly negative views of specific diagnoses following the reporting of high-profile cases in the media. For example, a general view exists that individuals with a diagnosis of **schizophrenia** are seen as dangerous to those around them in the United States and the UK (Hallam 2002; Pescosolido et al. 1999). Arguably this has been installed from news reports and dramatisations of individuals with this diagnosis. Research conducted by Koike et al. (2015) in Japan found that changing the name of schizophrenia helped to reduce the stigma. Although it is known that the media often portray a one-sided argument, this is not always recognised by the general population (Ashikali and Dittmar 2012).

Therefore, given the nature of stigma it can act as a barrier to mental health services, both initially in accessing them and engagement with them on an ongoing basis. In Case Study 9.4 Justine recognises how labelling impacted her sense of well-being.

CASE STUDY 9.4: LABELLING AND PTSD, JUSTINE'S STORY

I was diagnosed with PTSD over 15 years after an initial traumatic event, where I was attacked on the roadside at about 8 pm on a winter's evening by three men. I thought I was going to be killed or raped. Luckily they were disturbed so they suddenly ran off and I escaped. I then became a major witness in a high-profile murder trial and there was a lot of press coverage at the trial. I felt very guilty that I had not been able to identify them and that they were free on bail to murder the person who had been killed and this played out in my mind over and over. Immediately after the event I had panic attacks when going outside and I received counselling support from victim support.

I did at one stage avoid going outside and start to wonder if I had agoraphobia but I managed to overcome this by cycling rather than walking. For years I tried to put the event behind me and cope with work and my life, but my life seemed stuck – I had lots of bad dreams about being hunted or people trying to kill me and I had a series of difficult relationships, which was hard as I really wanted a family.

Eventually I started trying for a baby in my thirties. Years of infertility, miscarriages, surgeries and IVF followed and I eventually got pregnant with twins on what was to be my last attempt at IVF in my forties, but had pregnancy complications resulting in heavy bleeding through the pregnancy, premature delivery, sepsis and the twins needing intensive care and one needing surgery. When the anxiety symptoms started years later they were quite overwhelming, so I approached my GP who wanted to rule out hyperthyroidism. I think there was some initial disbelief from my GP that events some 15 years plus could be causing current physical symptoms, but this was overcome once the **community mental health team** wrote to my GP. It took five months to get the diagnosis and start a course of trauma-focused CBT and I was unable to work during this time.

The other issue I'd like to raise is around stigmatisation, of being labelled as having a mental illness. I feel very strongly that I have PTSD because of things that were done to me and happened to me and perhaps I wouldn't have become ill if life had been different. I think PTSD really needs to be viewed as psychological injury rather than mental illness and it's really helpful for victims' potential recovery for it to be viewed like this. Finally completing trauma therapy was really hard, but I now have a much better understanding of my condition and trauma and mental health issues in general, which I hope to bring into my professional life and work to provide learning opportunities for others.

Stigma may also act to prevent or delay access to social welfare, which can have an impact on an individual's basic needs being met, e.g. safe housing (Mojtabai 2010). Stigma also impacts on family members, **carers** and friends of the individual (Mandani et al. 2018; Upadhyay et al. 2016). While the consequences of stigma may not always be apparent, they are still present and it is essential that stigma is recognised and challenged at all levels of society (Koike et al. 2015; Pescosolido et al. 1999).

WHAT IS SOCIAL IDENTITY THEORY, STRUCTURAL STRAIN THEORY AND LABELLING THEORY?

Social identity theory

It is recognised that as part of cognitive processing, individuals recognise patterns, differentiate between objects, behaviours and situations as a function of survival. In a social context the identification of such patterns can lead to ingroups and outgroups.

(Continued)

(Continued)

Such categorisations allow recognition of other individuals and enable the application of mental constructs that provide direction during social interactions (Brown 2000).

Structural strain theory

This theory stipulates that society puts pressure on individuals to achieve, which could include measurable outputs such as wealth. This is based on meritocratic principles that the means to wealth is accessible to all in society. However, as Merton (1957) argues, the means to achieve are not fairly distributed and thus not accessible to all. Subsequently, strain occurs, which may lead individuals to access these through non-legal means. Such strain can be divided into two types:

Structural: societal level processes that impact 'top-down' on how the individual observes their needs.

Individual: the difficulties the individual experiences from attempting to identify the means to meet their needs.

Labelling theory

In a general context labelling theory explores how an individual's identity is influenced by the terms used to describe them. Here, deviance is not seen as being inherent to a specific action, rather it is a propensity for it to be labelled as a deviation from the norm (Becker 1963). In the context of mental health, through social interactions individuals may form beliefs about mental health, including the assessment and treatment of mental health difficulties. Such beliefs could relate to discrimination, unfairness and exclusion, for example, and inevitably can create difficulties for the individuals holding such beliefs, particularly if they encounter mental health difficulties themselves (Scheff 1966).

Emotional resilience

Definitions of emotional resilience are often linked to **psychological well-being**. Ryff (1989) proposed six components of well-being:

1. *Autonomy*: the capacity for self-determination.
2. *Environmental mastery*: the ability to manage one's surrounding world.
3. *Personal growth*: realisation of one's own potential.
4. *Positive relations with others*: having high-quality relationships.
5. *Purpose in life*: having meaning and direction in life.
6. *Self-acceptance*: having a positive self-regard.

Resilience is also the ability to successfully adapt to stress, to be flexible, hold inner strength and have the ability to bounce back and grow in the face of adversity (Sabir, Ramzan and Malik 2018). The resiliency model represents a conscious or unconscious choice individuals can take in response to the disruption of a stressor or adverse life event (see Figure 9.2).

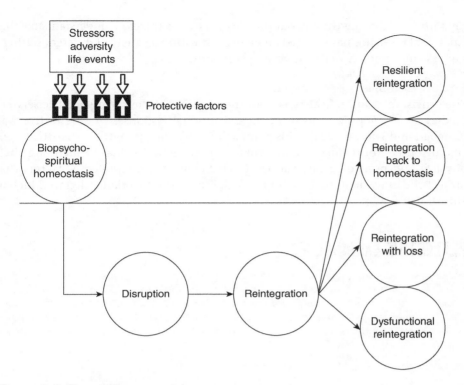

Figure 9.2 The resiliency model.

Source: Richardson (2002).

In the resiliency model resilient reintegration denotes growth and strength that occurs and bio-psycho-spiritual homeostasis refers to the 'adapted state of mind, body and spirit' (Richardson 2002, p. 311). Therefore, such disruption is an opportunity for growth and adaptation (Lavretsky 2014). Connected to this is the concept of post-traumatic growth, which relates to positive change that can occur following encounters with traumatic events (Manning-Jones, de Terte and Stephens 2015). Post-traumatic growth is defined as 'psychological growth following vicarious brushes with trauma' (Arnold et al. 2005, p. 243).

Therefore, it is recognised that emotional resilience requires the individual to be able to regulate their emotions by adapting their responses when the situation requires. It is stipulated that resilience isn't necessarily something we are born with, rather, it is formed as a result of secure attachments gained through interactions in the social world (Lavretsky 2014). By employing such strategies research has shown that an individual's experience can improve their psychological and physical well-being (Rauschenbach, Göritz and Hertel 2012). Indeed, resilience is often considered as a prerequisite for professionals working in the field of mental health and the wider health community (Frajo-Apor et al. 2016; Sabir et al. 2018). Interestingly, resilient individuals are also seen to have effective interpersonal relationships. Arguably, this leads to increased functioning in social settings, including work (Frajo-Apor et al. 2016). Lavretsky (2014) recognises resilience as being central to supporting well-being throughout the life course. It is therefore understandable that emotional resilience has received much interest within a variety of different settings, such as education, as well as in acute psychiatry.

Emotional resilience in therapy

The provision of dialectical behaviour therapy (DBT) in many psychiatric services focuses on developing tools to manage emotional responses in an effective way (Linehan and Dimeff 2001). This approach focuses on strengths rather than deficits, in other words, focusing on what enables the individual to maintain their physical and psychological well-being. This could be interpreted as factors that protect the individual, such as family, social support network or religion (Linehan and Dimeff 2001).

REFLECTIVE EXERCISE 9.2

Myles received a diagnosis of borderline personality disorder in his mid-twenties, after many years of being labelled as a troublemaker. He had been arrested by the police on many different occasions, usually for minor offences, although this appeared to escalate once he began using illegal drugs. He made an attempt to end his life after his mum died suddenly six months ago and he was admitted to an inpatient psychiatric ward for assessment and treatment.

Question: What might Myles learn from attending a DBT group?

Hint: Consider the coping strategies that DBT teaches.

CONCLUSION

It is evident that culture is an important part of understanding mental health difficulties and it is therefore essential that service providers facilitate culturally competent services. The individual's culture can have an impact on expression of symptoms, coping and support systems, in addition to accessing services for assessment and treatment. Equally the professional's culture plays an important role in the diagnosis and treatment models applied, as well as the way services are provided. Mental health difficulties are prevalent irrespective of cultural background, but given that culture is one of many factors that influence mental health difficulties it is essential that it is acknowledged. Thus the bio-psycho-social model is a useful framework to assess and treat the individual in a holistic manner (Engel 1980).

REFERENCES

American Psychiatric Association (1994) *The diagnostic and statistical manual of mental disorders* (4th ed.). Washington, DC: American Psychiatric Association.

Arnold, D., Calhoun, L. G., Tedeschi, R. G. and Cann, A. (2005) Vicarious posttraumatic growth in psychotherapy. *Journal of Humanistic Psychology* 45(2): 239–263.

Ashikali, E. and Dittmar, H. (2012) The effect of priming materialism on women's responses to thin-ideal media. *British Journal of Social Psychology* 51(4): 514–533.

Bassey, S. and Melluish, S. (2013) Cultural competency for mental health practitioners: a selective narrative review. *Counselling Psychology Quarterly* 26(2): 151–173.

Becker, H. S. (1963) *Outsiders: studies in the sociology of deviance*. London: Free Press of Glencoe.

Bennett, J., Kalathil, J. and Keating, F. (2007) *Race equality training in mental health services in England. Does one size fit all?* London: Sainsbury Centre for Mental Health.

Bhui, K. and Bhugra, D. (2007) Ethnic inequalities and cultural capability framework in mental healthcare. In K. Bhui and D. Bhugra (eds), *Textbook of cultural psychiatry* (pp. 81–92). Cambridge: Cambridge University Press.

Bozarth, J. (1998) Person-centred therapy: a revolutionary paradigm. Ross-on-Wye: PCCS Books.

Bronfenbrenner, U. (1979) *The ecology of human development: experiments by nature and design*. Cambridge, MA: Harvard University Press.

Bronfenbrenner, U. and Morris, P. (2006) The bioecological model of human development. In W. Damon and R. M. Lerner (eds), *Handbook of child psychology. Vol. 1: models of human-development* (6th ed., pp. 793–828). Hoboken, NJ: Wiley.

Brown, R. (2000) Social identity theory: past achievements, current problems and future challenges. *European Journal of Social Psychology* 30: 745–778.

Cross, T., Brazen, B., Dennis, K. and Isaacs, M. (1989) *Towards a culturally competent system of care*. Washington, DC: Georgetown University Child Development Center.

Davidson, L., Stayner, D. and Haglund, K. E. (1998) Phenomenological perspectives on the social functioning of people with schizophrenia. In K. T. Mueser and N. Tamer (eds), *Handbook of social functioning* (pp. 97–120). Boston, MA: Allyn & Bacon.

Department of Health (2003) *Inside/outside*. London: Department of Health.

DeVoe, E., Dondanville, K., Blankenship, A. and Hummel, V. (2018) PTSD intervention with military service member parents: a call for relational approaches. *Best Practice in Mental Health* 14(1): 40–53.

Dittmar, H. (2008) *Consumer culture, identity and well-being*. London: Psychology Press.

Engel, G. L. (1980) The clinical application of the biopsychosocial model. *American Journal of Psychiatry* 137(5): 535–544.

Frajo-Apor, B., Pardeller, S., Kemmler, G. and Hofer, A. (2016) Emotional intelligence and resilience in mental health professionals caring for patients with serious mental illness. *Psychology, Health and Medicine* 21(6): 755–761.

Fuertes, J., Stracuzzi, T., Bennett, J., Scheinholtz, J., Mislowack, A., Hersh, M. and Cheng, D. (2006) Therapist multicultural competency: a study of therapy dyads. *Psychotherapy: Theory, Research, Practice, Training* 43: 480–490.

Grabe, S., Ward, L. M. and Hyde, J. S. (2008) The role of the media in body image concerns among women: a meta-analysis of experimental and correlational studies. *Psychological Bulletin* 134: 460–476.

Groesz, L. M., Levine, M. P. and Murnen, S. K. (2002) The effect of experimental presentation of thin media images on body satisfaction: a meta-analytic review. *International Journal of Eating Disorders* 31: 1–16.

Hall, G., Iwamasa, G. and Smith, J. (2003) Ethical principles of the psychology profession and ethnic minority issues. In W. O'Donohue and K. Ferguson (eds), *Handbook of professional ethics for psychologists: Issues, questions, and controversies* (pp. 301–318). Thousand Oaks, CA: Sage.

Hallam, A. (2002) Media influences on mental health policy: long-term effects of the Clunis and Silcock cases. *International Review of Psychiatry* 14(1): 26–33.

Hofstede, G. H. (1991) *Cultures and organizations: software of the mind*. New York: McGraw-Hill.

Hunt, G. J. (1995) *Review of general psychiatry*. Norwalk, CT. Appleton & Lange.

Kawachi, I., Kennedy, B. P., Lochner, K. and Prothrow-Stith, D. (1997) Social capital, income inequality, and mortality. *American Journal of Public Health* 87: 1491–1498.

Kleinman, A. (1977) Depression, somatization and the 'new cross-cultural psychiatry'. *Social Science and Medicine* 11: 3–10.

Koike, S., Yamaguchi, S., Ojio, Y., Shimada, T., Watanabe, K. and Ando, S. (2015) Long-term effect of a name change for schizophrenia on reducing stigma. *Social Psychiatry and Psychiatric Epidemiology* 50(10): 1519–1526.

Lavretsky, H. (2014) *Resilience and aging: research and practice.* Baltimore, MD: Johns Hopkins University Press.

Lin, K. M. and Cheung, F. (1999) Mental health issues for Asian Americans. *Psychiatric Services* 50: 774–780.

Lin, N. (2001) *Social capital: a theory of social structure and action.* Cambridge: Cambridge University Press.

Linehan, M. M. and Dimeff, L. (2001) Dialectical behavior therapy in a nutshell. *The California Psychologist* 34: 10–13.

Lo, H. and Fung, K. (2003) Culturally competent psychotherapy. *Canadian Journal of Psychiatry* 48: 161–170.

Mandani, B., Ali Hosseini, S., Ali Hosseini, M., Noori, A. and Ardakani, M. (2018) Perception of family caregivers about barriers of leisure in care of individuals with chronic psychiatric disorders: a qualitative study. *Electronic Physician* 10(3): 6516–6526.

Manning-Jones, S., de Terte, I. and Stephens, C. (2015) Vicarious posttraumatic growth: a systematic literature review. *International Journal of Wellbeing* 5(2): 125–139.

Merton, R. K. (1957) *Social theory and social structure* (rev. ed.). New York: Free Press.

Mojtabai, R. (2010) Mental illness stigma and willingness to seek mental health care in the European Union. *Social Psychiatry and Psychiatric Epidemiology* 45(7): 705–712.

Pescosolido, B. A., Monahan, J., Link, B. G., Stueve, A. and Kikuzawa, S. (1999) The public's view of the competence, dangerousness, and need for legal coercion of persons with mental health problems. *American Journal of Public Health* 89: 1339–1345.

Pilgrim, D. (2011) Some limitations of the biopsychosocial model. *History and Philosophy of Psychology* 13(2): 17–23.

Pinder-Amaker, S. and Bell, C. (2012) A bioecological systems approach for navigating the college mental health crisis. *Harvard Review of Psychiatry* 20(4): 174–188.

Porter, R. (1997) *The greatest benefit to mankind: a medical history of humanity.* New York: Norton.

Rathod, S., Kingdon, D., Phiri, P. and Gobbi, M. (2010) Developing culturally sensitive cognitive behaviour therapy for psychosis for ethnic minority patients by exploration and incorporation of service users' and health professionals' views and opinions. *Behavioural and Cognitive Psychotherapy* 38: 511–533.

Rauschenbach, C., Göritz, A. and Hertel, G. (2012) Age stereotypes about emotional resilience at work. *Educational Gerontology* 38(8): 511–519.

Richardson, G. E. (2002) The metatheory of resilience and resiliency. *Journal of Clinical Psychology* 58(3): 307–321.

Ryff, C. D. (1989) Happiness is everything, or is it? Explorations on the meaning of psychological well-being. *Journal of Personality and Social Psychology* 57(6): 1069–1081.

Sabir, F., Ramzan, N. and Malik, F. (2018) Resilience, self-compassion, mindfulness and emotional well-being of doctors. *Indian Journal of Positive Psychology* 9(1): 55–59.

Scheff, T. J. (1966) *Being mentally ill: a sociological theory.* Chicago, IL: Aldine.

Shorter, E. (1997) *A history of psychiatry.* New York: Wiley.

Sue, D. W. and Sue, D. (1999) *Counseling the culturally different: theory and practice* (3rd ed.). New York: Wiley.

Taylor, S. M. and Dear, M. J. (1981) Scaling community attitudes toward the mentally ill. *Schizophrenia Bulletin* 7(2): 225–240.

Tseng, W. (2004) Culture and psychotherapy: Asian perspectives. *Journal of Mental Health* 13: 151–161.

Upadhyay, R., Srivastava, P., Singh, N. and Poddar, S. (2016) Community attitude and stigma towards mental illness: a gender perspective. *Journal of Psychosocial Research* 11(2): 335–341.

Wang, P. S., Berglund, P. and Kessler, R. C. (2000) Recent care of common mental disorders in the United States. *Journal of General Internal Medicine* 15: 284–292.

Webber M., Huxley P. and Harris T. (2011) Social capital and the course of depression: six-month prospective cohort study. *Journal of Affective Disorders* 129: 149–157.

Whaley, A. L. (1998) Issues of validity in empirical tests of stereotype threat theory. *American Psychologist* 5: 679–680.

Young, A. S., Klap, R., Shebourne, C. D. and Wells, K. B. (2001) The quality of care for depressive and anxiety disorders in the United States. *Archives of General Psychiatry* 58: 55–61.

10 INTERNATIONAL PERSPECTIVES ON MENTAL HEALTH

JO AUGUSTUS

LEARNING OBJECTIVES

After studying this chapter you will be able to:

- understand the global context of mental health service provision;
- identify the UK position in relation to international service provision;
- appreciate inequalities that exist at an international level;
- consider the future of global mental health communities.

INTRODUCTION

Mental health has increasingly become recognised as a key priority in international public health arenas. Most notably the World Health Organisation (WHO) highlighted the need for a comprehensive review of mental health services (WHO 2014). In the United Kingdom the Mental Health Service Reform highlighted mental well-being as a priority and looked at ways to improve the effectiveness of mental health services (Department of Health and Social Care 2013). The Global Burden of Disease study identified **depression** and **anxiety** disorders as contributing to the highest level of disability of all the mental health conditions (Whiteford et al. 2010). This is associated with the costs incurred in health care usage and absence from work (Katon et al. 2003; Simon et al. 1995). Olesen et al. (2012) quantified the total cost of mood disorders as €113.4 billion in Europe. In England it is noted that the cost of mental health difficulties is approximated as being 23% of the total cause of disability, which is much higher than chronic physical health conditions (Hewlett and Horner 2015; Richards et al. 2018).

One key international priority is associated with adolescence and young adults, predominantly as it is recognised that the emergence of mental health difficulties starts at this age (Van Droogenbroeck, Spruyt and Keppens 2018). Minas (2012) identifies key problem areas experienced by young adults globally, which include:

- high incidence of mental health difficulties (Kessler et al. 2007);
- rates of suicide in Asia (Levi, Vecchia and Saraceno 2003);
- reduced life expectancy of individuals with a diagnosis of **schizophrenia**;
- lower rates of employment and associated poverty (Lund et al. 2011);
- low- and middle-income countries with little or no access to mental health services.

Despite need being identified, research suggests that mental health has not been a priority for low- and middle-income countries (Saraceno et al. 2007; Saxena, Sharan and Saraceno 2003; Saxena et al. 2007).

If mental health problems are identified at an early stage in young adults, then interventions could help in the prevention of symptom deterioration. There is also a recognition that experiencing mental health difficulties from a young age can exacerbate or prolong its impact (Drake et al. 2012). Such impact can include **stigma** and discrimination, as well as social exclusion, which can act to worsen or maintain the mental health difficulty (Saxena et al. 2007; Thornicroft 2006). This can also cause delays in accessing education, career development and social skills. Therefore, the cost of mental health to society is significant and constitutes a large proportion of the global disease burden (Drake et al. 2012). It is recognised that effective interventions are available to support the **recovery** process, however, it is evident that difficulties exist in accessing services. Therefore, service provisions need to be reviewed to ensure that services are provided in a consistent and equitable way.

This chapter will explore the current context of mental health services and global evidence-based interventions that present an opportunity for international best practice. Many of the local or national issues raised will have implications and be applicable to the international context. The chapter aims to provide insight into the mental health systems of Sweden, Belgium, Germany, Argentina and China. These countries have been chosen as they are comparable to each other and to the UK, as they are all working towards the deinstitutionalisation of mental health service providers, albeit at different stages. As such it is hoped to provide the reader with insights into the possibilities of shared learning opportunities that can occur internationally.

The current context

Recent histories have been typified by socio-economic and political change. This includes the ending of the Cold War, European expansion, political tensions in the Middle East and most recently the War on Terror. Alongside this there has been an increasing movement of people, goods and services. While this presents opportunities for development it also could present challenges to providing effective and responsive services (Owen and Khalil 2007). Therefore, workforces need to be prepared to respond to diverse communities. In addition, the workforce is also diversifying in response to migration of professionals, perhaps practising in a different country to where they conducted their training. This could be typified by a shortage in recruiting and retaining nursing staff (Lu, White and Barriball 2008). Therefore, a twofold response is needed to support both staff and service users in understanding the factors that will influence the presentation of mental health issues (Minas and Cohen 2007). Akin to this is the need to challenge discrimination, value diversity and create a flexible societal structure that can support the ever-changing landscape of mental health recovery (Owen and Khalil 2007).

During the latter part of the twentieth century in Western Europe there was a shift away from committing individuals with mental health problems to asylums, towards community services (Bergmark, Bejerholm and Markström 2017; Fawcett and Karban 2005; Goodwin 1997). This largely resulted from a recognition that asylum provisions were costly and not consistently fit for purpose and also due to advancements made in medicine (Knapp et al. 2007). Deinstitutionalisation shifted the emphasis of care provision to the outpatient community services. Despite the reduction in the number of available beds, there remains a need for inpatient care. However, rather than focusing on long-term institutionalisation, these services work towards recovery and rehabilitation (Becker and Kilian 2006; Samele, Frew and Urquía 2013), which include assessment and regular reviews with a focus on reintegration into the community. Therefore, a move towards the development of integrated care systems was born (Bergmark et al. 2017; Knapp et al. 2007).

Alongside such service shifts, policy has also shifted towards **social inclusion**, through challenging stigma, shared decision-making and involvement of multi-agencies, for example. As a consequence, individualised care planning is now a standard approach, offering evidence-based interventions (Slade 2009). This approach is established in the UK and Germany and more recently was adopted in Sweden (Bergmark et al. 2017). Although arguably this has caused a shift in emphasis away from community as an aid to recovery to the individual and therefore the balance needs to continually be readdressed.

GLOBAL MENTAL HEALTH PROVISION

Sweden

Sweden has a generous welfare system for all its residents, funded and provided for predominantly by the public sector. This approach is recognised as the Nordic welfare model, which promotes equality and access to services that are comprehensive, of high-quality and available to all (Kvist and Greve 2011) and includes a large amount of resources available for mental health. Sweden is known for its soft approach to strategy and associations to community interest. Here there exists a paradox as, on the one hand, the government has to take a top-down approach to policy, while on the other hand, allow for flexible implementation locally. However, research is lacking on the impact of such government approaches on the outcomes of individuals accessing mental health services (Bergmark et al. 2017). Meeting the needs of the local service user with directives from central government often presents challenges. The Swedish government policies that focus on community mental health services clearly promote the provision of psycho-social interventions.

There have been three key documents presented to the Swedish government that reflected a clear shift towards the provision of evidence-based interventions. The third document, in 2012, identified clear action plans in the delivery of psycho-social interventions and was clearly underpinned by the first two documents in 1994 and 2009 (see Table 10.1).

Table 10.1 Three key policy documents that support the provision of community mental health service provision in Sweden

	Document A (1994)	Document B (2009)	Document C (2012)
Objectives	Improve individuals' lives and participation in society	Knowledge-based care of good quality that fits people's needs	Care based on equality, safety, accessibility and good quality
Desired characteristics of psycho-social interventions	Scientifically tested methods Knowledge from psychiatry	Based on evidence, high competence, experience, and individual adaption	Based on best available knowledge, implementation of evidence-based practice
Named psycho-social interventions discussed	Not discussed (except the experimental activity) Personal representative	Personal representative	Personal representative, assertive community, treatment, and case managers
Governing strategies	Changes in legislation Stimulus grants to support development	Changes in legislation Stimulus grants, steering document, regulation agreements	Guidelines, systematic reviews, performance-based grants
Governance	Relatively autonomous state	Mix of the state's responsibilities and mobilisation of others	High degree of networking strategies. 'Steering not rowing'
Strategies for managing political risk	Shotgun Agencies have a high level of discretion	Shotgun Clarification of the government's role as stimulator and auditor	Shotgun Highlighting own efforts and other's responsibilities 'Delegated networking'

These interventions provided a whole-person approach and included areas such as housing. Specialist integrated teams prioritised groups such as children and those with **severe and enduring mental difficulties** and included supporting individuals with mental health difficulties integrate into society. To promote such an approach the government has implemented media campaigns and financial incentive as well as including public opinion in decision-making (Bergmark et al. 2017).

Community-based interventions that have been undertaken in the last four years have included support for families and **carers**, as well as the use of web-based interventions to improve access. For example, a web-based mindfulness programme aimed at promoting the well-being of families of individuals with mental health difficulties (Elgán et al. 2016; Stjernswärd and Hansson 2017) and the provision of psycho-education for individuals, families and carers (Liljeroos et al. 2017; Svensson and Hansson 2014). Interestingly, the terms the Swedish government used to describe individuals with mental health difficulties have shifted to 'people with ill health', perhaps reflecting a move towards anti-discriminatory practice. As such, Sweden is often highlighted as offering a high standard of mental health service provision and a model that other countries can aspire to.

Belgium

In the move to community-based care, the Belgium government and local providers have placed emphasis on the importance of continuity of services in the provision of care (Durbin et al. 2006). Disruptions in continuity have led to poor outcome measures, including deterioration of symptoms (Lorant et al. 2016). The mental health service delivery reform encouraged the involvement of service networks, e.g. partnerships (Nicaise, Dubois and Lorant 2014). Lorant et al. (2016) highlight Belgium's health care system as having three key characteristics:

1. The health care system is organised as a regulated system.
2. The health care system is fragmented.
3. Prior to reform, policy deinstitutionalisation was incomplete.

Although local autonomy is promoted, health authorities are more tightly governed. There is also the expectation of health insurance, which in turn could create unequal access to services. Service fragmentation could create barriers to collaborative working processes. Finally, there are geographic variations in the services provided. The mental health service reform is founded on the creation of networks between mental health services, enabling the provision of comprehensive care. This was underpinned by aims to strengthen the structure of community care, with the processes of care coordination to improve patient outcomes (see Figure 10.1). Such an approach provides services aimed at a holistic or whole-person approach, including intensive inpatient psychiatric programmes, housing provision and prevention programmes embedded in **primary care** (Lorant et al. 2016).

In current research health promotion features as an intervention used to promote a whole-person approach. For example, strategies to improve physical health care in mental health care provision (Verhaeghe et al. 2013). This was evident in findings of an intervention based on motivational interviewing that reduced weight gain and anxiety in obese pregnant women (Bogaerts et al. 2013). Deplus et al. (2016) conducted a small-scale study that highlighted the potential of using mindfulness as an intervention to improve emotional regulation in adolescence.

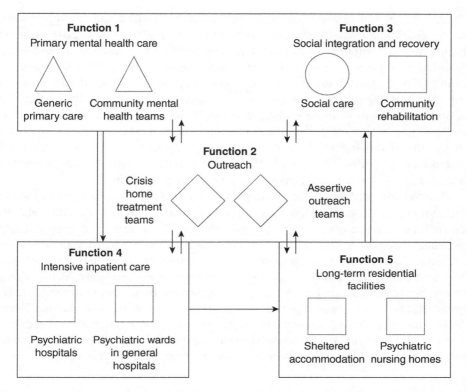

Figure 10.1 Overview of the Belgian mental health delivery system. The five basic care functionalities suggested by the reform blueprint are represented with the type of services mainly involved in the implementation of these functionalities. Triangles represent services mainly organised at the regional level; squares represent services mainly organised at the federal level; circles represent services mainly organised at the local level; and diamonds represent the newly established mobile teams.

Source: Lorant et al. (2016).

Germany

Psychiatric care in Germany is largely provided by inpatient and outpatient units as well as psychiatrists and psychologists working in office-based settings. A variety of psycho-social interventions are also provided in community and residential settings, including occupational support (Salize, Rossler and Becker 2007). There are regional differences in the service provision as mental health services are funded from different sources, e.g. statutory and private medical insurance. Therefore, supporting the transition of individuals moving from inpatient to outpatient psychiatric services could be disrupted if systems are not aligned. This presents an opportunity to integrate services through a reform, adopting a bio-psycho-social approach in the assessment and treatment of mental health difficulties based in the community. Mental health care services could then be improved by moving away from inpatient services and moving towards the development of outpatient service provision

(Becker, Kilian and Kosters 2016; Karow et al. 2012), but in doing so support structures need to be established in the community. Valentini et al.'s (2016) research highlighted the importance of providing interventions to reduce carer burden and maintain continuity of care for individuals with mental health difficulties. Hajek and König's (2016) research supports this through recognising the importance of providing resources to support the provision of intergeneration caregiving. Such an approach would need to be evaluated in order for future recommendations to be made. There is also the recognition of developing an evidence base in support of promoting well-being in those of working age, through the use of creative arts (Martin et al. 2018). Again, with all emerging evidence bases future research is required to support the recommendation of their continuation.

The Network for Mental Health project was developed in 2009 by a private medical insurance company and brought together local mental health services. This collaboration of services was intended to provide support for a variety of mental health difficulties, prevent inpatient stay and move towards a needs-based approach in the community. This project was accepted by other insurance companies and evaluated. Mueller-Stierlin et al. (2017) compared the patient outcomes for individuals engaging in the Network for Mental Health project to those receiving treatment as usual. The results showed no difference in outcomes, however, the Network for Mental Health project had significant improvement in patient satisfaction and their perception of participating in treatment. Therefore, the project presented a number of considerations to take forward to future developments in mental health service provision.

Argentina

There is a recognition that psychiatric services in Argentina remain focused on asylums alongside community care provisions (Ardila-Gýmez et al. 2014). The wider health services are seen as being fragmented (Saguinetti et al. 2016). A reform that began in 2010 and subsequent delays were partly attributed to the dictatorship between 1976 and 1983, when community services were dissolved. Such service closure was largely due to suspicion of their function and perception of threat to the dictatorship. During the dictatorship there were reports of political violence, part of which was the systematic and forced disappearance of individuals (Crenzel 2011).

One example of a recent psychiatric community service is the 'assisted discharge and rehabilitation programme', established in 1999 to support individuals who have been hospitalised for long periods (Ardila-Gýmez 2014). Basic needs are addressed including the provision of accommodation and skills taught to enable the individual to function in a state-supported local community setting (Goffman 1961). Integration continues through attendance at educational programmes and the continuation of such services depends on the resources available to enable individuals to continue to live in the community. It is hoped that such assisted discharge programmes will be offered across Argentina (Ardila-Gýmez 2014). In addition, Carlos et al. (2016) place emphasis on the importance of reviewing both societal characteristics and mental health services, in order to support the development of community-based services and also encourage further integration of physical and mental health services.

Interestingly, Rausch Herscovici et al. (2013) noted that the dominant therapeutic provision in Argentina is a psychodynamic psychotherapeutic approach. This is seen to originate from prominent psychoanalyst migrants who settled in Argentina during the Second World War. However, there is movement towards evidence-based interventions that can be integrated with psychodynamic approaches. This could be seen to reflect a shift towards individualised diagnosis and specific therapeutic approaches. A move towards systems supporting mental health is also apparent, for example community interventions designed to support families. Here psychoanalysis is increasingly being recognised as one therapeutic approach, rather than the dominant one (Rausch Herscovici et al. 2013). In addition, research conducted by Saguinetti et al. (2016) reported that community- and home-based mental health provisions improved access, increased adherence to the programmes and also patient satisfaction when compared to inpatient treatment programmes.

China

Since the China reform in 1978, there have been clear changes in family structure and a shift away from the nuclear extended family to those living alone or as a couple. There has also been a movement of the populous from rural to urban centres (Yao et al. 2017). China is a large country, with over 50 ethnic groups and makes up approximately 18% of the world's population. China plays an important role in global economic development and governance (Xie 2017). Its reform of social governance is significant to the provision of health care, including mental health services. Mental health service reform began in China in 2005, although the geographic variations in China create some complexity in the design of health care systems (Xie 2010, 2013). There is a recognition that the development of mental health services has been delayed due to the stigma and discrimination often associated with mental health in China. New mental health law was established in 2013 and the National Mental Health Work Plan (2015–2020) acknowledged three stages of development that included (Xie 2017):

- improvement of specialist services;
- integration with community services;
- improvement of organisation at a societal level.

The provision of specialist training for doctors across China underpinned the establishment of psychiatric services. Such services are centred on psychiatric hospitals, although community-based provision developed post-2005 reform and has significantly advanced since 2015 (Liu et al. 2011; Ma et al. 2012). The new plan focuses on developing sustainable services based on need and identifies specific areas of mental health to focus on, e.g. suicide prevention, severe and enduring mental health disorders and interventions for disasters. There is also emphasis on integration of services, promotion of mental health across the life course as well as standardisation of treatment interventions (Xie 2017).

   Yao et al.'s (2017) research measured family function through the use of the APGAR (adaptation, partnership, growth, affection and resolve) scale. The results showed that improved family function improved mental health, therefore reinforcing the need to involve family in the development of services. Ma et al.'s (2012) research showed dropout rates were low in an integrated hospital community provision, where psychoeducation was provided to families of individuals with a diagnosis of psychosis. Research conducted by Jie et al. (2015) found that a developed knowledge base improved the attitude towards individuals with mental health difficulties in community-based services. This highlights a need to develop training programmes for professionals involved in community-based initiatives that focus on the needs of the local population. This was supported by research conducted by Wu et al. (2017), highlighting the need for improving mental health literacy through training for the general population of China in order to improve support for individuals with mental health difficulties.

CONCLUSION

Global communities and social change

It is evident from this chapter that despite the socio-political variations in the countries explored, there exists much similarity in mental health service provision and research findings. For example, across all countries it was recognised that deinstitutionalisation and the development of **community mental health teams** is a complex process with barriers operating at different levels of governance. Varying levels of integration between inpatient and community-based services was evident, perhaps reflected in the stage of reform in which the country is positioned. In addition, while the importance of inpatient settings is known, the efficacy of recovery is increasingly seen in integrated community services. Here the roles of the family, carer and community are central to the recovery of the individual. Ways to challenge discrimination and prejudice is acknowledged as pertinent, however in many countries such constructs about mental health continue to create barriers. The use of evidence-based practice is used to develop the provision of bio-psycho-social interventions, with emphasis on the psycho-social.

Bergmark et al. (2017) mention the use of guidelines for community services, alongside the use of action plans for the provision of specific evidence-based interventions as Sweden advocates. Initiatives focusing on inclusive approaches that involve shared working with service users, professionals, families, carers and members of the wider community are evident. Such an alliance of public health groups work alongside government policy in the wider international community. Social change is happening at varying paces worldwide and there exists much opportunity to create global communities with the aim of supporting shared learning. A general consensus from the countries explored in this chapter appear to advocate for contemporary mental health care to provide inclusive, integrated and responsive mental health services, provided by multi-professionals (Mueller-Stierlin et al. 2017).

REFERENCES

Ardila-Gýmez, S. (2014) Users' perspective on the evaluation of mental health services. *International Journal of Mental Health* 43(2): 70–80.

Becker, T. and Kilian, R. (2006) Psychiatric services for people with severe mental illness across Western Europe: what can be generalized from current knowledge about differences in provision, costs and outcomes of mental health care? *Acta Psychiatrica Scandinavica* 113: 9–16.

Becker, T., Kilian, R. and Kosters, M. (2016) Policies, guideline implementation and practice change: how can the process be understood? *Epidemiology and Psychiatric Sciences* 26(2): 115–118.

Bergmark, M., Bejerholm, U. and Markström, U. (2017) Policy changes in community mental health: interventions and strategies used in Sweden over 20 years. *Social Policy and Administration* 51(1): 95–113.

Bogaerts, A., Devlieger, R., Nuyts, E., Witters, I., Gyselaers, W. and Van den Bergh, B (2013) Effects of lifestyle intervention in obese pregnant women on gestational weight gain and mental health: a randomized controlled trial. *International Journal of Obesity* 37(6): 814–821.

Crenzel, E. (2011) Between the voices of the state and the human rights movement: never again and the memories of the disappeared in Argentina. *Journal of Social History* 44(4): 1063–1076.

Department of Health and Social Care (2013) *2010 to 2015 government policy: mental health service reform.* www.gov.uk/government/publications/2010-to-2015-govern ment-policy-mental-health-service-reform/2010-to-2015-government-policy-mental-health-service-reform (accessed 24 May 2018)

Deplus, S., Billieux, J., Scharff, C. and Philippot, P. (2016) A mindfulness-based group intervention for enhancing self-regulation of emotion in late childhood and adolescence: a pilot study. *International Journal of Mental Health and Addiction* 14(5): 775–790.

Drake, R., Bond, G., Thornicroft, G., Knapp, M. and Goldman, H. (2012) Mental health disability: an international perspective. *Journal of Disability Policy Studies* 23(2): 110–120.

Durbin, J., Goering, P., Streiner, D. L. and Pink, G. (2006) Does systems integration affect continuity of mental health care? *Administration and Policy in Mental Health* 33(6): 705–717.

Elgán, T., Kartengren, N., Strandberg, A., Ingemarson, M., Hansson, H., Zetterlind, U. and Gripenberg, J. (2016) A web-based group course intervention for 15–25-year-olds whose parents have substance use problems or mental illness: study protocol for a randomized controlled trial. *BMC Public Health* 16(1): 1–8.

Fawcett, B. and Karban, K. (2005) *Contemporary theory, policy and practice in mental health.* London: Routledge.

Goffman, E. (1961) *Asylums: essays on the social situation of mental patients and other inmates.* New York: Random House.

Goodwin, S. (1997) *Comparative mental health policy: from institutional to community care.* London: Sage.

Hajek, A. and König, H. (2016) The effect of intra- and intergenerational caregiving on subjective well-being: evidence of a population based longitudinal study among older adults in Germany. *Plos ONE* 11(2): 1–11.

Hewlett, E. and Horner, K. (2015) *Mental health analysis profiles (MhAPs).* London: OECD Publishing.

Jie, L., Juan, L., Thornicroft, G., Hui, Y., Wen, C. and Yuanguang, H. (2015) Training community mental health staff in Guangzhou, China: evaluation of the effect of a new training model. *BMC Psychiatry* 15: 1–10.

Karow, A., Reimer, J., König, H. H., Heider, D., Bock, T., Huber, C., Schöttle, D., Mesiter, K., Rietschel, L., Ohm, G., Schulz, H., Naber, D., Schimmelmann, B. G. and Lambert, M. (2012) Cost-effectiveness of 12-month therapeutic assertive community treatment as part of integrated care versus standard care in patients with schizophrenia treated with quetiapine immediate release (ACCESS trial). *Journal of Clinical Psychiatry* 73: e402–e408.

Katon, W. J., Lin, E., Russo, J. and Unützer, J. (2003) Increased medical costs of a population-based sample of depressed elderly patients. *Archive of General Psychiatry* 60(9): 897–903.

Kessler, R. C., Angermeyer, M., Anthony, J. C., De Graaf, R., Demyttenaere, K., Gasquet, I., De Girolamo, G., Gluzman, S., Gureje, O., Haro, J. M., Kawakami, N.,

Karam, A., Levinson, D., Medina Mora, M. E., Oakley Browne, M. A., Posada-Villa, J., Stein, D. J., Adley Tsang, C. H., Aguillar-Gazoia, S., Alonso, J., Lee, S., Heeringa, S., Pennell, B. E., Berglund, P., Gruber, M. J., Petukhova, M., Chatterji, S. and Ustün, T. B. (2007) Lifetime prevalence and age-of-onset distributions of mental disorders in the World Health Organization's World Mental Health Survey Initiative. *World Psychiatry* 6: 168–176.

Knapp, M., McDaid, D., Mossialos, E. and Thornicroft, G. (2007), *Mental health policy and practice across Europe: the future direction of mental health care*. Maidenhead: Open University Press.

Kvist, J. and Greve, B. (2011) Has the Nordic welfare model been transformed, *Social Policy and Administration* 45(2): 146–160.

Levi, F., La Vecchia, C. and Saraceno, B. (2003) Global suicide rates. *European Journal of Public Health* 13: 97–98.

Liljeroos, M., Ågren, S., Jaarsma, T., Årestedt, K., Strömberg, A., Ågren, S., Årestedt, K. and Strömberg, A. (2017) Long-term effects of a dyadic psycho-educational intervention on caregiver burden and morbidity in partners of patients with heart failure: a randomized controlled trial. *Quality of Life Research*, 26(2): 367–379.

Liu, J., Ma, H., He, Y. L., Xie, B., Xu, Y. F., Tang, H. Y. et al. (2011) Mental health system in China: history, recent service reform and future challenges. *World Psychiatry* 10(3): 210–216.

Lorant, V., Grard, A., Van Audenhove, C., Helmer, E., Vanderhaegen, J. and Nicaise, P. (2016) Assessment of the priority target group of mental health service networks within a nation-wide reform of adult psychiatry in Belgium. *BMC Health Services Research* 16: 1–9.

Lu, H., While, A. and Barriball, K. (2008) Job satisfaction among nurses: a literature review. *International Journal of Nursing Studies* 42: 211–227.

Lund, C., De Silva, M., Plagerson, S., Cooper, S., Chisholm, D., Das, J., Knapp, M. and Patel, V. (2011) Poverty and mental disorders: breaking the cycle in low-income and middle-income countries. *Lancet* 378: 1502–1514.

Ma, N., Liu, J., Wang, X., Gan, Y., Ma, H., Ng, C., Jia, F. and Yu, X. (2012) Treatment dropout of patients in the National Continuing Management and Intervention Program for Psychoses in Guangdong Province from 2006 to 2009: implications for mental health service reform in China. *Asia-Pacific Psychiatry* 4(3): 181–188.

Martin, L., Oepen, R., Bauer, K., Nottensteiner, A., Mergheim, K., Gruber, H. and Koch, S. (2018) Creative arts interventions for stress management and prevention: a systematic review. *Behavioral Sciences* 8(2): 1–18.

Minas, H. (2012) The Centre for International Mental Health Approach to Mental Health System Development. *Harvard Review of Psychiatry* 20(1): 37–46.

Minas, H. and Cohen, A. (2007) Why focus on mental health systems? *International Journal of Mental Health Systems* 1: 1.

Mueller-Stierlin, A., Helmbrecht, M., Herder, K., Prinz, S., Rosenfeld, N., Walendzik, J., Holzmann, M., Dinc, U., Schützwohl, M., Becker, T. and Kilian, R. (2017) Does one size really fit all? The effectiveness of a non-diagnosis-specific integrated mental health care program in Germany in a prospective, parallel-group controlled multi-centre trial. *BMC Psychiatry* 17: 1–12.

Nicaise, P., Dubois, V. and Lorant, V. (2014) Mental health care delivery system reform in Belgium: the challenge of achieving deinstitutionalisation whilst addressing fragmentation of care at the same time. *Health Policy* 115(2): 120–127.

Olesen, J., Gustavsson, A., Svensson, M., Wittchen, H. U. and Jonsson, B. (2012) The economic cost of brain disorders. *Europe. European Journal of Neurology* 19(1): 155–162.

Owen, S. and Kahill, E. (2007) Addressing diversity in mental health care: a review of guidance documents. *International Journal of Nursing Studies* 44(3): 467–478.

Rausch Herscovici, C., Campos González, S., Label, H., Zevallos Vega, R. and Chong García, N. (2013) Development and practice of the systems paradigm in

Argentina, Chile and Peru. *Contemporary Family Therapy: An International Journal* 35(2): 200–211.

Richards, D., Duffy, D., Blackburn, B., Earley, C., Enrique, A., Palacios, J., Franklin, M., Clarke, G., Sollesse, S., Connell, S. and Timulak, L. (2018) Digital IAPT: the effectiveness and cost-effectiveness of internet-delivered interventions for depression and anxiety disorders in the Improving Access to Psychological Therapies programme: study protocol for a randomised control trial. *BMC Psychiatry* 18: 1.

Saguinetti, C., Marin, G., Herrera, N., Molteni, O., Milito, S., Molinero, C., Posse, A., Riquelme, J., Rodriguez, M., Amadeo, J., Belauzaran, L., Cejas, N., Gonzalez, O. M., Kess, G., Lòpez N. and Maestropiedra, M. (2016) Mental health in Argentina: interdisciplinary program based in community care. *Contemporary Behaviour in Health Care* 2(1): 41–43.

Salize, H. J., Rossler, W. and Becker, T. (2007) Mental health care in Germany: current state and trends. *European Archives of Psychiatry and Clinical Neurosciences* 257: 92–103.

Samele, C., Frew, S. and Urquía, N. (2013) *Mental health systems in the European Union member states, status of mental health in populations and benefits to be expected from investments into mental health: European profile of prevention and promotion of mental health (EuroPoPP-MH)*. Nottingham: Institute of Mental Health and the European Commission.

Saraceno, B., van Ommeren, M., Batniji, R., Cohen, A., Guereje, O., Mahoney, J., Sridhar, D. and Underhill, C. (2007) Barriers to improvement of mental health services in low-income and middle-income countries. *Lancet* 370: 1164–1174.

Saxena, S., Sharan, P. and Saraceno, B. (2003) Budget and financing of mental health services: baseline information on 89 countries from WHO's project atlas. *Journal of Mental Health Policy Economics* 6: 135–143.

Saxena, S., Thornicroft, G., Knapp, M. and Whiteford, H. (2007) Resources for mental health: scarcity, inequity, and inefficiency. *Lancet* 370: 878–889.

Simon, G., Ormel, J., VonKorff, M. and Barlow, W. (1995) Health care costs associated with depressive and anxiety disorders in primary care. *American Journal of Psychiatry* 152(3): 352–357.

Slade, M. (2009) *Personal recovery and mental illness: a guide for mental health professionals*. Cambridge: Cambridge University Press.

Stjernswärd, S. and Hansson, L. (2017) User value and usability of a web-based mindfulness intervention for families living with mental health problems. *Health and Social Care in the Community* 25(2): 700–709.

Svensson, B. and Hansson, L. (2014) Effectiveness of mental health first aid training in Sweden: a randomized controlled trial with a six-month and two-year follow-up. *Plos ONE* 9(6): 1–8.

Thornicroft, G. (2006). *Shunned: discrimination against people with mental illness*. Oxford: Oxford University Press.

Valentini, J., Ruppert, D., Magez, J., Stegbauer, C., Bramesfeld, A. and Goetz, K. (2016) Integrated care in German mental health services as benefit for relatives: a qualitative study. *BMC Psychiatry* 16: 1–9.

Van Droogenbroeck, F., Spruyt, B. and Keppens, G. (2018) Gender differences in mental health problems among adolescents and the role of social support: results from the Belgian health interview surveys 2008 and 2013. *BMC Psychiatry* 18: 1–9.

Verhaeghe, N., Clays, E., Vereecken, C., De Maeseneer, J., Maes, L., Van Heeringen, C., De Bacquer, D. and Annemans, L. (2013) Health promotion in individuals with mental disorders: a cluster preference randomized controlled trial. *BMC Public Health* 13(1): 1–14.

Whiteford, H. A., Degenhardt, L., Rehm, J., Baxter, A. J., Ferrari, A. J., Erskine, H. E., Charlson, F. J., Norman, R. E., Flaxman, A. D., Johns, N., Burstein, R., Murray, C. J. and Vos, T. (2013) Global burden of disease attributable to mental and substance use disorders: findings from the global burden of disease study 2010. *Lancet* 382(9904): 1575–1586.

WHO (2014) *Mental health action plan 2013–2020*. Geneva, Switzerland: World Health Organisation.

Wu, Q., Luo, X., Chen, S., Qi, C., Long, J., Xiong, Y., Liao, Y. and Liu, T. (2017) Mental health literacy survey of non-mental health professionals in six general hospitals in Hunan Province of China. *Plos ONE* 12(7): 1–13.

Xie, B. (2010) Challenges and major legislation solution for mental health in China. *Shanghai Arch Psychiatry* 22(4): 193–199.

Xie, B. (2013) Experience and lessons draw from the process of mental health legislation in China. *Zhongguo Xin Li Wei Sheng Za Zhi* 27(4): 245–248.

Xie, B. (2017) Strategic mental health planning and its practice in China: retrospect and prospect. *Shanghai Archives of Psychiatry* 29(2): 115–119.

Yao, C., Liuyi, Z., Fang, W., Ping, Z., Beizhu, Y. and Yuan, L (2017) The effects of family structure and function on mental health during China's transition: a cross-sectional analysis. *BMC Family Practice* 18: 1–8.

GLOSSARY

Anxiety Anxiety disorders range from mild to severe worry, fear or immobilising terror. They can be characterised by physical symptoms such as racing heart or feeling fidgety or restless. Most people experience anxiety at some point in their lives and some nervousness in anticipation of a real situation, e.g. a job interview. However, if a person's everyday life is significantly impacted, such as by avoidance of everyday activities, this could be related to an anxiety disorder. Anxiety can also be associated with depression.

Approved mental health professional (AMHP) A social worker or other professional approved by a local authority to carry out a variety of functions under the Mental Health Act.

Behavioural therapy Focuses on managing unwanted behaviours through rewards, reinforcements, and desensitisation. Desensitisation, or exposure therapy, is a process of confronting something that causes anxiety, discomfort, or fear and overcoming the unwanted responses. Behavioural therapy often involves working with others, especially family and close friends, to reinforce a desired behaviour.

Bipolar disorder Characterised by extreme mood swings with recurrent episodes of depression and mania marked by periods of the individual's usual behaviour. Bipolar disorder is known to be genetic and typically begins in the mid-twenties and continues throughout life. Without treatment, people who have bipolar disorder often go through devastating life events such as relationship difficulties, loss of job or career, substance abuse and suicide.

Capacity The ability to take a decision about a particular matter at the time the decision needs to be made. Some people may lack capacity to take a particular decision (e.g. to consent to treatment) because they cannot understand, retain, use or weigh the information relevant to the decision. A legal definition of lack of capacity for people aged 16 or over is set out in section 2 of the Mental Capacity Act 2005. *See also* consent.

Care Programme Approach (CPA) A system of care and support for individuals with complex needs, which includes an assessment, a care plan and a care coordinator. It is used mainly for adults in England who receive specialist mental health care. There are similar systems for supporting other groups of individuals including children and young people (children's assessment framework or CAF), older adults (single assessment process) and people with learning disabilities (person-centred planning).

Carer Someone who helps another person, usually a relative or friend, in their day-to-day life unpaid. This is not the same as someone who provides care professionally, or through a voluntary organisation.

Child and adolescent mental health services (CAMHS) Specialist mental health services for children and adolescents. CAMHS covers all types of provision and intervention from mental health promotion and primary prevention, specialist community-based services through to very specialist care as provided by inpatient units for children and young people with mental illness. It is mainly composed of a multidisciplinary workforce with specialist training in child and adolescent mental health.

Chronic health condition A long-term condition that an individual lives with, which may often fluctuate and for which there is usually no cure such as diabetes, asthma or some mental health problems.

Clinical Commissioning Group (CCG) The NHS body responsible for commissioning (arranging) NHS services for a particular part of England from NHS trusts, NHS foundation trusts and independent sector providers. CCGs replaced primary care trusts from 1 April 2013. CCGs' commissioning plans are reviewed by the NHS Commissioning Board (NHS England). CCGs are generally responsible for commissioning mental health care, except for specialist care commissioned by the NHS Commissioning Board.

Cognitive behavioural therapy (CBT) A combination of cognitive and behavioural therapies, this approach helps people change negative thought patterns, beliefs and behaviours so they can manage symptoms and enjoy the life they want to lead.

Cognitive therapy (CT) Aims to identify and correct distorted thinking patterns that can lead to feelings and behaviours that may be causing the individual difficulty, be self-defeating or even self-destructive. The goal is to replace such thinking with a more balanced view that, in turn, leads to more fulfilling and productive behaviour.

Community mental health team (CMHT) A team of mental health workers who work together in a community setting. They often include psychiatrists, community psychiatric nurses, occupational therapists, social workers, care workers and psychologists.

Community treatment order (CTO) The legal authority for the discharge of a patient from detention in hospital, subject to the possibility of recall to hospital for further medical treatment if necessary. Community patients are expected to comply with the conditions specified in the community treatment order.

Consent Agreeing to allow someone else to do something to or for you. Particularly consent to treatment. Valid consent requires that the person has the capacity to make the decision (or the competence to consent, if a child), and they are given the information they need to make the decision, and that they are not under any duress or inappropriate pressure.

Consultant In a hospital a consultant refers to a specially trained doctor who has finished his training and works in one area of medicine, usually with a team of doctors in training and other professionals working with them. In other areas of work, a consultant is someone who is consulted in order to get his opinion on something.

Counsellors (also known as psychotherapists) Counsellors work in various settings such as the independent or voluntary sector, GP surgeries and hospitals. Counsellors offer counselling to those in need, drawing on a variety of therapeutic models depending on their training and experience. Counsellors aim to identify the problems a person is facing in any sphere of life and to help them discover effective ways of dealing with these. Talking through a problem with somebody neutral can often help a person to see a way forward.

Crisis resolution and home treatment (CRHT) Short-term, round-the-clock help provided in a non-hospital setting during a crisis. The purpose of this care is to avoid inpatient hospitalisation, help stabilise the individual and determine the next appropriate step.

Dementia Significant loss of intellectual abilities such as memory capacity, severe enough to interfere with social or occupational functioning. Dementia is a neurological condition that makes it hard for a person to remember, learn and communicate. Diagnostic criteria also include impairment of attention, orientation, memory, judgement, language, motor and spatial skills and function. This disorder can also affect a person's mood and personality. This may eventually lead to them being unable to care for themselves.

Depression A mood disorder characterised by intense feelings of sadness, loss of pleasure and enjoyment, which persist beyond a few weeks. It is associated with many physical symptoms such as disturbance of sleep, appetite, and concentration. Depressed people often feel tired, guilty and can find normal life extremely difficult. Depression can be associated with anxiety.

Deprivation of Liberty Safeguards (DoLS) The framework of safeguards under the Mental Capacity Act 2005, as amended by the Mental Health Act 2007, for people who need to be deprived of their liberty in their best interests for care or treatment to which they lack the capacity to consent themselves.

Early intervention A process used to recognise warning signs for mental health problems and to take early action against factors that put individuals at risk. Early intervention can help people get better in less time and can prevent problems from becoming worse.

Electroconvulsive therapy (ECT) A form of medical treatment for mental disorder in which a small, carefully controlled electric current is introduced into the brain. It is administered in conjunction with a general anaesthetic and muscle relaxant medications and is occasionally used to treat very severe depression.

Empowerment Giving people the skills, knowledge attitudes and power to allow or enable them to be more responsible for their own lives, health and care.

Equality Act 2010 A law making it unlawful (either directly or indirectly) to discriminate against a person on the basis of a protected characteristic (as defined in the Act). Imposes a public sector equality duty on public bodies.

Evidence based An intervention based on widely accepted evidence formed from research. This evidence can be from scientific studies (e.g. a randomised controlled trial) or based on the collective experience of senior professionals. Such evidence can be used to develop guidelines to help health care workers improve the care they provide.

Hallucinations Experiences of sensations that have no known source. Some examples of hallucinations include hearing non-existent voices, seeing non-existent things and experiencing pain sensations with no physical cause.

Holding powers The powers in section 5 of the Mental Health Act 2007, which allow hospital inpatients to be detained temporarily so that a decision can be made about whether an application for detention should be made. There are two holding powers. Under section 5(2) doctors and approved clinicians can detain patients for up to 72 hours. Under section 5(4), certain nurses can detain patients for up to 6 hours.

Independent mental health advocate (IMHA) An advocate available to offer help to patients under arrangements that are specifically required to be made under the Mental Health Act.

Mania A symptom of bipolar disorder characterised by exaggerated excitement, physical overactivity and profuse and rapidly changing ideas that may be scattered or tangential thoughts. A person in a manic state feels an emotional high and generally follows their impulses or urges, which may put them at risk of harm to themselves or others.

Mental health A state of emotional well-being in which an individual is able to use his or her thinking and feeling abilities, live with others and meet the ordinary demands of everyday life.

Mental illness or ill-health A state where the person's mental health is disrupted so that their thinking, emotions or behaviour are affected to an extent that it has an effect on their daily life. However, it is important to note this does not necessarily mean they will have a mental health diagnosis.

Multidisciplinary team (MDT) A professional team including staff from a range of different professions.

Obsessive-compulsive disorder (OCD) A chronic anxiety disorder characterised by recurrent and unwanted thoughts or rituals. The obsessions and the need to perform rituals can take over a person's life if left untreated. They feel they cannot control these thoughts or rituals.

Occupational therapists (OTs) An occupational therapist can have many different roles. They help people to adapt to their environment and to cope with their daily life. OTs may work in hospitals or in the community. They assess a person's ability to look after themselves, e.g. self-care, cooking and housework. They plan interventions that involve occupations that are meaningful to the person. This may be done in purpose-built occupational therapy departments in hospitals or in the patient's own home. OTs work with both individuals and groups. They can set goals for individuals with depression to encourage them to achieve more than they have been able to do while ill. They may get patients involved in specific job-related training schemes to improve their decision-making and planning about the future. Group work is often aimed at increasing people's social interactions.

Panic disorders People with panic disorder experience terror that happens suddenly and without warning. Typified by a racing heart, individuals often describe themselves as being in flight or freeze mode. This can lead to persistent worry that a panic attack could overcome them at any moment, e.g. a fear of panic.

Paranoia Symptoms of paranoia include feelings of persecution and an exaggerated sense of self-importance. The disorder is present in many mental health problems and it is rare as an isolated mental illness. A person with paranoia can usually work and function in everyday life since the delusions involve only one area, although their lives can be isolated and limited.

Person-centred care The patient is at the centre of their diagnosis and treatment. Patient-centred care seeks an integrated vision of the patient's world, finds common ground and creates a shared management plan, enhancing health promotion and providing a therapeutic relationship with professionals. Patient-centred care is therefore based on the patient's problems, needs, feelings and beliefs.

Practitioner A person who practices a specific profession. They may be regulated by a professional body that enables them to provide health care services.

Primary care Community services that provide open access to patients. They include GPs, pharmacists, dentists, district nurses and health visitors and many others. Also called Tier 1 services.

Psychological well-being A state of being characterised by health, happiness and prosperity. It is a broader term than mental health and includes the wider aspects of a person's life, not just how they feel.

Recovery Does not always mean cure, rather it includes management of symptoms, improved quality of life and the ability of the individual to lead the life they want to lead. Mental health recovery is a journey enabling a person with a mental health problem to live a meaningful life of his or her choice while striving to achieve his or her full potential.

Schizophrenia A mental health diagnosis characterised by psychotic symptoms that include delusions, hallucinations and disordered thinking that may be apparent from a person's fragmented, disconnected and sometimes nonsensical speech. Other symptoms may include social withdrawal, poor motivation and the absence of emotional expression.

Secondary care Specialist health services that are usually hospital based and serve a wide geographical area. Aside from accident and emergency services, they are usually accessed through a referral from a primary care professional.

Service provider A person or an organisation that provides a service to a member of the public. This can be an NHS body, a small local group or a national voluntary sector organisation.

Severe and enduring mental difficulties The term used to describe a group of illnesses that can cause more severe mental health problems. It includes schizophrenia, bipolar affective disorder (manic depression) and other psychotic illnesses that on occasion have a significant impact on all aspects of the individual's functioning.

Social inclusion Ensures that marginalised individuals and those living in poverty have greater participation in decision-making, which affects their lives, allowing them to improve their living standards and their overall well-being.

Stigma Discrimination based upon social constructs surrounding mental health difficulties. It may cause individuals to be marginalised or mistreated and therefore lead to social isolation and health inequalities.

Voluntary sector (sometimes called the third sector) This sector is diverse, ranging from small local groups staffed exclusively by volunteers, to large national charities. They are not established for financial gain and re-invest any surpluses to further their primary objectives.

INDEX